Table of Contents

DC:0-5™

Diagnostic Classification of Mental Health and Developmental Disorders of Infancy and Early Childhood

VERSION 2.0

ZERO TO THREE

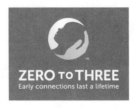

Washington, DC

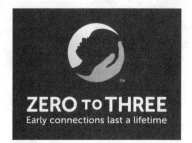

Published by

ZERO TO THREE
(202) 638-1144
Toll-free orders (800) 899-4301
Fax: (202) 638-0851
Web: www.zerotothree.org

10 9 8 7 6 5 4 3 2
ISBN 978-1-938558-70-2
Printed in the United States of America

Suggested citation: ZERO TO THREE. (2021). *DC:0–5™: Diagnostic classification of mental health and developmental disorders of infancy and early childhood* (Version 2.0). Washington, DC: Author. (Original work published 2016)

Preface

DC:0–5: Diagnostic Classification of Mental Health and Developmental Disorders of Infancy and Early Childhood (DC:0–5™) is a welcome and much-awaited guide for diagnosing mental disorders in early childhood. Users will find it incorporates the best available general knowledge from research, clinical practice, and early child development. Why "much-awaited"? As the Chair of the former DC:0-3R system which this supersedes, I can say that phrase with conviction because our general knowledge about identifying and intervening with early childhood disorders has been growing at a fast pace, and major change has been needed. In this light, the Introduction to DC:0–5 is a must-read for users, explaining how the Diagnostic Classification system has evolved in response to needs, and continues to evolve.

The reader will find that major changes include not only the identification of new evidence-based syndromes, but also a needed inclusion of the 3–5 year age period. Further, there is as an increased emphasis on users appreciating and documenting contexts for diagnostic classification, which is so important for early childhood development. The latter fact leads the designers of DC:0–5 to retain the multi-axial system, in order to supplement the clinical diagnoses of Axis I. In addition to the relational context of Axis II, these include the contexts of physical health conditions, psychosocial stressors, and developmental competence (in Axes II–V).

Another major change worth mentioning at the outset has to do with the importance of early caregiving relationships. Compelling recent evidence from research indicates that infant and early child attachments and their disorders are relationship specific; a fact that justifies the inclusion of a relationship specific disorder among the Clinical Disorders of Axis I. Additionally, a much-expanded section on Relational Context in Axis II is included that states "understanding the relationship context should be included in every assessment of infants and young children." Accordingly, users are provided with a rating scheme of "strength," "not a concern," or "concern" for dimensions of relationship functioning for one or more primary caregiver relationships (in Part A) and for the broader caregiving environment (in Part B). The latter is designed to include the understanding of co-parenting, sibling, and other important relationships in the child's development.

In this preface, it seems important to remember what diagnostic classification is and what it is not. Diagnostic classification is for professional communications, linking to general knowledge about disorders, derived from research and clinical practice. It is descriptive of syndromes and symptoms involving distress and the impairment of functioning over time. A system of diagnostic classification is not a "textbook," or worse yet a "bible" for clinicians or others to use, as has sometimes been portrayed. And as clinicians know, they are classifying disorders, not individuals. For individuals, it is a major task of the clinician to use a system of diagnostic classification as one significant step in the further process of *diagnostic formulation*. This involves applying the general knowledge of disorder classification to a developing individual in the particulars of living, with the formulation of an opinion about the needs for further assessment (or not) and plans for further intervention (or not). It involves careful history taking in caretaker interviews, direct observations, clinical empathy, and holistic judgments in which patterns of child behavior and experience are taken into account. Again, although DC:0–5 may provide more general information about the assessment of context in its Axes of II–V than other classification systems, it does not provide a guide or a manual for clinical formulation.

DC:0–5 is not intended to compete with the diagnostic classifications of the *Diagnostic and Statistical Manual of Mental Disorders* (5th ed.; DSM; American Psychiatric Association, 2013) or the International Classification of Diseases (ICD; 10th ed.; World Health Organization, 1992). It arises because current versions of the latter do not adequately cover syndromes in the earliest postnatal years—syndromes that clinicians encounter and may require urgent attention and preventative interventions. While it is the case that some early childhood syndromes may link to knowledge about pathways of etiology, in other instances, where there is insufficient evidence, they may not and yet may still point to needed interventions as well as research. And it is important to keep in mind that this is during a time in development when accumulating evidence shows that early adaptive experience and its disruptions and adversities have profound influences on development throughout the lifespan. Additionally, non-competition is emphasized by the provision within DC:0–5 for suggested possible "crosswalks" for classifications of DC:0–5 to current DSM-5 and ICD-10 classifications of disorder, and by the stated intention that in the future infancy and early childhood disorders be included within the DSM and ICD systems.

As noted, general knowledge about diagnostic classification in infancy and early childhood is *evolving* and DC:0–5 has made substantial changes that reflect that. Accordingly, there are new complexities, new criteria, new terms, and new issues. Current users of DC:0–3R may wonder about what resources are available beyond the current publication for help in questions about understanding and implementation. It is helpful to know that the ZERO TO THREE website, www.zerotothree.org, is a significant resource that may be consulted for additional information about usage.

Robert N. Emde, MD
Professor of Psychiatry, Emeritus, University of Colorado School of Medicine

Acknowledgments

The Diagnostic Classification Revision Task Force gratefully acknowledges the help given to us by the global community of infant and early childhood mental health professionals who responded to our requests for information and feedback during the many stages of the revision process. More than 10 years after the publication of the *Diagnostic Classification of Mental Health and Developmental Disorders of Infancy and Early Childhood, Revised Edition* (DC:0–3R; ZERO TO THREE, 2005), hundreds of individuals and many groups gave us valuable advice that reflected the wisdom of their experience. These respondents are obviously committed to advancing clinical work with infants/young children and their families by updating diagnostic classification through specifying criteria that are based on up-to-date knowledge and evidence. We have hope for the future because of this community's compassion and commitment to the most vulnerable infants/young children and their families worldwide.

We are extremely grateful to the individuals (890 professionals from six continents) who responded to the DC:0–3R Revision Survey in 2013. Respondents included clinicians from a range of disciplines as well as those involved in research and administration in the infant mental health field. In May 2015, and again in October 2015, we posted proposed revisions in the diagnostic criteria for public comment. We also hosted public input forums at the ZERO TO THREE National Training Institutes in 2013 and 2015, and at the World Association of Infant Mental Health Congress in Edinburgh, Scotland, in 2014. We are grateful to the many individuals who provided expert feedback.

Special thanks are due to the individuals who served as consultants to the Diagnostic Classification Revision Task Force. They conducted literature reviews and provided crucial feedback. We are grateful to Kimberly Carpenter, Lauren Franz, Sherika Hill, Kathryn Humphreys, Ivy Giserman Kiss, Shirley Poyau, and Timothy Soto.

Several individuals deserve special acknowledgment for their constructive contributions throughout the process. Their invaluable feedback guided our efforts. We are grateful to Thomas Anders, Marianne Barton, Zeynep Biringen, Karen Burstein, Irene Chatoor, Roseanne Clark, Annette Copa, Robert Emde, Gil Foley, Janna Hack, Kathleen Hipke, Barbara Howard, Lucy Hudson, Maria Kroupina, Julie Larrieu, Claire Lerner, Connie Lillas, Karlen Lyons-Ruth, James McHale, Lucy Miller, Pia Risholm Mothander, Angela Narayan,

Ruth Paris, Jen Perfetti, Julie Ribaudo, Michelle Sarche, Michael Scheeringa, Rebecca Shahmoon-Shanok, Arietta Slade, Richard Stedman, Raymond Sturner, Linda Tuchman-Ginsberg, Suzi Tortora, Lauren Wakschlag, Rachel Bryant Waugh, Serena Weider, Catherine Wright, and Paula Zeanah.

Without the support of ZERO TO THREE, its Executive Director, Matthew Melmed, and its Executive Committee, the creation of *DC:0–5: Diagnostic Classification of Mental Health and Developmental Disorders of Infancy and Early Childhood* (DC:0–5™) would never have been accomplished.

We owe a great deal of gratitude to the Revision Task Force that created DC:0–3R (chaired by Robert Emde) and to the original Task Force that constructed the *Diagnostic Classification of Mental Health and Developmental Disorders of Infancy and Early Childhood* (DC:0–3; ZERO TO THREE, 1994; co-chaired by Stanley Greenspan and Serena Wieder). The members of these groups are acknowledged in Appendix C. DC:0–5 is the product and legacy of their pioneering work.

Lastly, we extend thanks to the infants/young children and families who have taught us all so much.

Diagnostic Classification Revision Task Force

Charles H. Zeanah, Chair
Alice Carter
Julie Cohen
Helen Egger
Mary Margaret Gleason
Miri Keren
Alicia Lieberman
Kathleen Mulrooney
Cindy Oser

Robert Emde, Special Advisor

Introduction

The *DC:0–5: Diagnostic Classification of Mental Health and Developmental Disorders of Infancy and Early Childhood* (DC:0–5™) represents an effort to update and expand previous versions of a nosology of infancy/early childhood disorders: *Diagnostic Classification of Mental Health and Developmental Disorders of Infancy and Early Childhood* (DC:0–3; ZERO TO THREE, 1994) and *Diagnostic Classification of Mental Health and Developmental Disorders of Infancy and Early Childhood, Revised Edition* (DC:0–3R; ZERO TO THREE, 2005). The Diagnostic Classification Revision Task Force of ZERO TO THREE spent more than 3 years on this revision; updating the manual was a meticulous process that took into account emerging empirical evidence and advances in theoretical and clinical understandings. Other nosologies are available for mental health and developmental disorders, of course, including the *Diagnostic and Statistical Manual of Mental Disorders* (5th ed.; DSM–5; American Psychiatric Association, 2013) and the *International Classification of Diseases* (10th ed.; ICD–10; World Health Organization, 1992). Nevertheless, neither of these alternatives is ideally suited to consider the clinical definitions of disorders of infancy/early childhood.

There is no question that the empirical base of disorders in infants/young children lags behind what is known about disorders in older children, adolescents, and adults. Nevertheless, an increasing number of studies, including some epidemiologic and longitudinal studies, have been conducted with infants/young children. In preparing this nosology, the Task Force drew heavily on this empirical base. Of course, as with all nosologies, the strength of the empirical background varies from disorder to disorder.

In addition, clinical experience was used to shape and refine criteria. After surveying 20,000 clinicians worldwide about DC:0–3R in 2013, the Task Force received 890 completed surveys from practitioners on six continents with many comments about disorders and axes. In addition, preliminary criteria for disorders were posted on the ZERO TO THREE website in May 2015 and in October 2015, and input was solicited about those early drafts. The collective clinical experiences of Task Force members also were included in determining the definitions of the DC:0–5 disorders.

We approached our task atheoretically, with the goal of providing descriptive criteria that lend themselves to assessments of reliability and validity and minimizing the need for unsupported inferences or attributions beyond what is clinically observable. We agreed that all aspects of the nosology, even including the multiaxial approach, would be reviewed before inclusion. Because of the special importance of context for infants'/young children's development, all five axes from DC:0–3 and DC:0–3R were retained, although most have been extensively revised and updated. Axis I defines disorders but each axis contributes to the clinical formulation.

Please note: We respect each infant, toddler, and young child. However, for brevity, the term "infant/young child" is used throughout this book.

A Summary of Changes From DC:0–3R to DC:0–5

Initial reviews of the literature, new data, and practitioner input, as well as discussions of the Task Force, made it clear that the revision of DC:0–3R would be extensive. Many of the differences that distinguish DC:0–5 from DC:0–3R specify and clarify criteria for the classification categories already designated in Axis I. Several new disorders have been added to Axis I, whereas others that were in DC:0–3R have been excluded. Changes in DC:0–5 include the following:

- The new edition includes disorders occurring in infants/young children through 5 years old; the new title DC:0–5 reflects this change.

- The Task Force made an effort to be more comprehensive in defining disorders rather than referring clinicians to other nosologies if the disorders were not included in the nosology. Thus, other well-known disorders in infants/young children, such as Autism Spectrum Disorder and Attention Deficit Hyperactivity Disorder, have been included.

- In Axis I, the disorders are clustered into sections that group similar disorders together.

- Each disorder includes a diagnostic algorithm to clarify how the criteria are to be used with a goal of maximizing interrater reliability.

- Age limitations and duration criteria have been included when appropriate.

- Almost every disorder includes text that describes what is known about the clinical presentations, course, and correlates.

- In an effort to discern true disorders from transient behaviors or individual differences, every disorder includes distress or functional impairment as a criterion.

- DC:0–5 defines criteria for several new disorders, including Early Atypical Autism Spectrum Disorder, Inhibition to Novelty Disorder, Disorder of Dysregulated Anger and Aggression of Early Childhood, and Relationship Specific Disorder of Infancy/Early Childhood.

- A new Sensory Processing Disorders section has been added and includes Sensory Over-Responsivity Disorder, Sensory Under-Responsivity Disorder, and Other Sensory Processing Disorder.

- "Feeding Behavior Disorders" have been renamed "Eating Disorders of Infancy/Early Childhood" to focus the attention on the infant's/young child's contribution to an activity that is necessarily interactive and that universally occurs within the context of a relationship. The number of defined disorders in this category has been substantially reduced and clustered into broader categories of Overeating Disorder, Undereating Disorder, and Atypical Eating Disorder.

- Numerical codes for DC:0–5 Clinical Disorders are provided to facilitate inclusion of DC:0–5 disorders in health care delivery and electronic medical records. Numerical coding provides consistency among various disorder lists and can prevent misunderstanding when translating diagnosis into other languages.

- Links to the corresponding DSM–5 and ICD–10 disorders are included in the text for each DC:0–5 Axis I disorder.

- Extensive revisions have been made to Axis II (Relational Context). The axis now includes two parts: a rating of the level of adaptation of the primary caregiving relationship(s) and a rating of the level of adaptation of the caregiving environment—that is, the broader family relational network (including coparenting) in which the infant/young child is developing.

- Axis III has been expanded to include illustrative examples of medical conditions that should be noted.

- Axis IV has maintained the Psychosocial and Environmental Stressors Checklist but has added categories and some specific stressors.

- Axis V has been extensively revised to focus on developmental competencies that integrate domains of emotional, social-relational, language-social communication, cognitive, and movement and physical development. A table of "Developmental Milestones and Competency Ratings" is included in Appendix A to aid practitioners.

- For each disorder, links are included between DC:0–5, DSM, and ICD codes. A complete crosswalk of all DC:0–5 disorders is available at www.zerotothree.org/dc05resources

A History of ZERO TO THREE's Diagnostic Classification Efforts

DC:0–3, which was published in 1994 by ZERO TO THREE, was created to address the significant need for a systematic, developmentally based approach to the classification of mental health and developmental difficulties in the first 4 years of life (i.e., birth through 3 years old). The design and formation of DC:0–3 represented the first effort by a group of expert and extremely experienced clinicians to devise a useful scheme that would complement, but not replace, other approaches to diagnostic classification systems for older children and adults, such as the *Diagnostic and Statistical Manual of Mental Disorders* (4th ed.;

DSM-IV; American Psychiatric Association, 1994) and the ICD–10. The creators of DC:0–3 sought to take note of new knowledge concerning (1) factors that contribute to adaptive and maladaptive patterns of development and (2) the meaning of individual differences in infancy (ZERO TO THREE, 2005). Their goal was to develop classification criteria that could improve professional communication, clinical formulation, and research. The revised DC:0–3, published in 2005 as DC:0–3R, was created more than a decade after the publication of the original diagnostic classification system. The new manual provided a revision that updated criteria for classifications, included new knowledge from clinical experience, and provided clarification for areas of continued ambiguity. The current revision/update of DC:0–3R, DC:0–5, captures new findings pertinent to diagnosis in infants/young children, updates criteria for classifications, introduces several new disorders, expands the age range from birth through 3 years old to birth through 5 years old, substantially revises the axes, and tackles unresolved concerns in the field since DC:0–3R was published in 2005.

The Origins of DC:0–3

Note: *This section is replicated in its entirety from DC:0–3R (ZERO TO THREE, 2005).*

DC:0–3 was the product of a multidisciplinary Diagnostic Classification Task Force that was established in 1987 by ZERO TO THREE: National Center for Infants, Toddlers, and Families, an organization representing interdisciplinary professional leadership in the field of infant development and mental health. Task Force members included clinicians and researchers from infant mental health centers throughout North America and Europe. Members of the group systemically analyzed case reports from participating centers, identified recurring patterns of behavioral problems, and described categories of disorders. The process was an open one, in which opinions were sought from a variety of disciplines.

Through expert consensus, an initial set of diagnostic categories emerged. Task Force members recognized that, given the limitations of infant mental health knowledge, diagnostic categories in the new classification system could only be descriptive—that is, representative of meaningful symptom patterns. Sometimes categorical descriptions included associated events (e.g., between a traumatic event and a group of symptoms) or developmental features (e.g., between sensory or motor patterns and a group of symptoms seen at a particular stage of early development). The result was a scheme based on five axes:

- Axis I: Primary Diagnosis
- Axis II: Relationship Disorder Classification
- Axis III: Medical and Developmental Disorders and Conditions
- Axis IV: Psychosocial Stressors
- Axis V: Functional Emotional Developmental Level

Having accomplished this, the Task Force recognized that this new guide for diagnostic classification of mental disorders in this age group would be tentative. Wording from the Introduction to DC:0–3 is instructive.

In any scientific enterprise, but particularly in a new field, a healthy tension exists between the desire to analyze findings from systematic research before offering even initial conceptualizations and the need to disseminate preliminary conceptualizations so they can serve as a basis for collecting systematic data, which can lead to more empirically based efforts... The development of DC:0–3 represents an important first step: the presentation of expert, consensus-based categorizations of mental health and developmental disorders in the early years of life... It is an initial guide for clinicians and researchers to facilitate clinical diagnosis and planning, as well as communication and further research (p. 11).

The Origins of DC:0–3R

In 2002, a revision to DC:0–3 was proposed, and in 2003, ZERO TO THREE selected and appointed a Revision Task Force. The group was tasked with drafting a revised version of DC:0–3, providing needed specifications and clarifications of criteria to allow reliability among clinicians and to advance the evidence-based evolution of the system (ZERO TO THREE, 2005). For 2 years, the group considered clinical literature and other diagnostic systems, developed and disseminated two surveys to DC:0–3 users worldwide, and gathered draft language and comments from experts across disciplines. The Task Force communicated each week (via conference calls and in person) to hone text and diagnostic criteria.

The revised DC:0–3, published in 2005 as DC:0–3R, drew on empirical research and clinical practice that had occurred worldwide since the 1994 publication and extended the depth and criteria of DC:0–3. DC:0–3R supported clinicians in diagnosing and treating mental health problems in the first years of life. It also encouraged readers to consult with the DSM–IV–TR (4th ed., text rev.; DSM–IV–TR; American Psychiatric Association, 2000) and the ICD–10; both manuals describe some of the mental health disorders that are usually first diagnosed in the early years.

DC:0–3 had presented a decision tree that implied that an infant/young child would have a single diagnosis. In DC:0–3R, the decision tree was maintained with regard to the infant's/young child's "primary diagnosis," but it also emphasized that more than one diagnosis was possible. The inclusion of comorbidity was a significant change in emphasis from DC:0–3.

DC:0–3R continued the multiaxial classification system that had been so valuable in clinical formulation. The labels for the DC:0–3R axes were almost the same as those in DC:0–3, with just a few slight changes in wording as recommended by users:

- Axis I: Clinical Disorders
- Axis II: Relationship Classification
- Axis III: Medical and Developmental Disorders and Conditions
- Axis IV: Psychosocial Stressors
- Axis V: Emotional and Social Functioning

DC:0–3R provided a common language that allowed professionals across disciplines—clinicians, researchers, faculty, and policy makers—to communicate accurately and effectively with each other (via the DC:0–3R crosswalks) and to link clinical knowledge about infant/early childhood disorders.

The Usefulness of DC:0–3R and the Need for Revision

Clinicians who address the mental health needs of infants/young children found DC:0–3R to be a useful nosology. It was well received by clinicians from around the world; in addition to the original English edition, translations have been published in several languages including Dutch, French, Italian, Japanese, Korean, Polish, and Romanian.

Despite its widespread use, the Task Force members who authored DC:0–3R were aware that it would need to be updated. Although it represented the best thinking at the time, the authors noted that at some future time, the collected experience with DC:0–3R, as well as additional new issues and studies, would necessitate a new edition. There were several key reasons that DC:0–3R needed to be revised and updated. First, by 2016, more than a decade had passed since DC:0–3R was published; substantial research on infancy/early childhood psychopathology has been published during that time. Second, the decision to revise and update DC:0–3R coincided with the publication of DSM–5. Although DSM–5 made an intentional effort to be more developmentally sensitive, it did not sufficiently capture the range of disorders characteristically seen in infancy/early childhood. Finally, there were some unresolved issues in the field since DC:0–3R was published that could be addressed with the benefit of a decade of clinicians' experiences in using it.

In 2013, ZERO TO THREE appointed the Diagnostic Classification Revision Task Force to draft a revised and updated version of DC:0–3R within 3 years. The Task Force studied clinical literature and other diagnostic systems, developed and disseminated a DC:0–3R survey of users worldwide, posted criteria for public comment, and gathered draft language and feedback from world-renowned experts who represented a variety of professional disciplines. The Task Force communicated on a biweekly basis via conference calls and met in person several times a year to develop diagnostic criteria and to draft and hone text. DC:0–5 is the product of this 3-year effort. Details of the revision process are presented in Appendix B.

Assessment, Diagnosis, and Formulation

Note: The following section was modified from a similar section in DC:0–3R (ZERO TO THREE, 2005).

Assessment is the result of gathering information from review of records, obtaining history from caregivers, and conducting informal and more structured observations of behavior. *Diagnosis* is the identification and classification of specific infant/young child disorders. *Formulation* is the way in which the infant's/young child's clinical presentation is understood in the context of the infant's/young child's relationships, biology, social network, and developmental status. A formulation can guide a treatment plan by highlighting the risk and protective factors, identifying those that are modifiable, and prioritizing clinical factors amenable to treatment.

For the practicing clinician, the assessment process is ongoing. One does not make a diagnosis on the basis of a onetime "snapshot" of symptoms, but rather, one collects information about the infant's/young child's behavior over time to understand multiple aspects of presenting problems as well as variations in adaptation and development that reveal themselves on different occasions and in different contexts. Axes II–V are useful in characterizing the context of Axis I symptoms and disorders.

We assess individuals, but we classify disorders. The primary purpose of classification of disorders is so that professionals—including clinicians, researchers, and policy makers—can communicate clearly about descriptive syndromes. Having a shared and standard nosology allows clinicians to link their observations to a growing body of knowledge concerning etiology, pathogenesis, the course of a disorder, and expectations concerning treatment. Using the common language of a diagnostic classification system facilitates the connection of individuals to existing services and thus can aid in the mobilization of appropriate systems of mental health care.

DC:0–5 reflects research that has demonstrated that comorbidity in infants/young children is not only possible, it is common. Furthermore, as with older children and adolescents, infants/young children with two or more disorders are more likely to have elevated impairment in their functioning compared with infants/young children with only one disorder.

In discussing clinical formulation with respect to infants/young children, the authors of DC:0–3 made two key observations:

- Assessment and diagnostic classification are guided by the awareness that all infants/young children have their own developmental progression and show individual differences in their motor, sensory, language, cognitive, affective, and interactive patterns.

- All infants/young children are participants in relationships. Infants'/young children's most significant relationships are usually those within the family. Families, in turn, participate in relationships within their larger communities and cultures.

Any intervention or treatment program should be based on as complete an understanding of the infant/young child and the infant's/young child's relationships as is possible to achieve. Pressed for time, clinicians may be tempted to focus attention on a limited number of variables while giving only cursory regard to other influences on development. Clinicians may also be tempted to avoid assessing those areas of an infant's/young child's functioning where the constructs or research tools are not fully developed or where gaps in their own training exist. Although these temptations are understandable, any clinician or clinical team who is responsible for making a complete diagnostic assessment of an infant/young child and planning an appropriate intervention program must take into account all relevant areas of the infant's/young child's functioning. Independently or with a team of colleagues, the clinician is obliged to apply state-of-the-art knowledge to each area of functioning and to evaluate both strengths and weaknesses in the infant/young child and family.

A clinician or team needs a number of sessions to understand how an infant/young child is developing in each area of functioning. A few questions to parents or caregivers about each area may be appropriate for screening but not for a full evaluation. A comprehensive evaluation usually requires a minimum of 3–5 sessions of 45 or more minutes each. A complete evaluation will typically involve the following:

- Interviewing the parent(s) about the infant's/young child's developmental and medical history;

- Directly observing family functioning (e.g., family and parental dynamics, the caregiver–infant/young child relationship, and interaction patterns);

- Gaining information, through direct observation and report, about the infant's/young child's individual characteristics, language, cognition, social reciprocity, and affective and behavioral expression; and

- Assessing sensory reactivity and processing, motor tone, and motor planning capacities.

In addition to consideration of clinical disorders, findings from a comprehensive evaluation should lead to preliminary notions about the following:

- The nature of the infant's/young child's pattern of strengths and difficulties, including the level of overall adaptive capacity and functioning in the major areas of development (emotional, social-relational, language-social communication, cognitive, and movement and physical) in comparison with age and culturally expected developmental patterns;

- The relative contribution to the infant's/young child's competencies and difficulties of the different areas assessed (e.g., family relationships, interactive patterns, stress, and constitutional–maturational patterns); and

- A comprehensive treatment or preventive intervention plan to deal with the first and second points above.

DC:0–5 continues the multiaxial classification system that has been useful in clinical formulation. Use of the multiaxial system for clinical formulation focuses the clinician's attention on the factors that may be contributing to the difficulties of the infant/young child, adaptive strengths, and additional areas of functioning in which intervention may be needed. Two of the labels for DC:0–5's axes are the same as those in DC:0–3R; however, the labels for the other three axes have been revised and updated. All of the axes have been revised substantially:

- Axis I: Clinical Disorders
- Axis II: Relational Context
- Axis III: Physical Health Conditions and Considerations
- Axis IV: Psychosocial Stressors
- Axis V: Developmental Competence

Cultural Considerations in Diagnosing Disorders in Infants/Young Children

Infants'/young children's behavior and expression of emotion are shaped from the moment they are born by family cultural values and practices that are often unconsciously held but that carry enormous power as parameters of what is right and wrong in raising an infant/young child. These values and practices imbue every aspect of caregiving, from concrete decisions, such as where and with whom the baby sleeps and when to start toilet training, to adult expectations about what the infant/young child is allowed or not allowed to say and do in different situations. For these reasons, diagnosing an infant/young child who is experiencing mental health problems must include developing an understanding and appreciation of the family's cultural background and the parents' socioeconomic conditions, national origin and history, immigration status, ethnic and racial identity, sexual orientation, religious and spiritual practices, and other sources of diversity.

The accuracy and usefulness of the diagnostic process are significantly enhanced when clinicians actively elicit parents' perceptions and causal explanations for the infant's/young child's mental health problems, and when clinicians inform themselves about the possible cultural influences shaping parents' views. The importance is particularly evident when the family and the clinician are from different cultural backgrounds and may not be familiar with each other's prevailing attitudes and beliefs about accepted child-rearing practices, but it is also necessary to avoid false assumptions of shared beliefs when clinicians come from a similar background. Given the growing cultural diversity of most societies, learning about the specific values and practices of the infant's/young child's family is now a central component of best clinical practice. In this sense, cultural sensitivity and cultural competence should be considered integral elements of clinical sensitivity and clinical competence.

Learning to incorporate cultural considerations into the diagnostic process is a long-term effort because cultural groups are more often than not characterized by internal heterogeneity within the group, and families are becoming increasingly multicultural. For example, people from the same race may differ in ethnicity, religion, socioeconomic status, educational attainment, and many other factors, and family members may have different demographic characteristics. In addition, individuals often see themselves as having several identities simultaneously because of the different prisms of the groups to which they belong. Cultural considerations must honor the dynamic nature of cultures as well as the individual family members' complex adaptations to the multiple contexts in which they operate.

In assessing an infant/young child, it is useful to keep in mind that mainstream clinical attitudes and practices in the field of infancy/early childhood mental health are shaped by professional assumptions that may not be shared by the family. A clinician's view of what is normative or healthy may be in conflict with the family's views of what is right and wrong—for example, in terms of the young child's curiosity about the body and emerging sexual exploration or the young child's expression of anger at parents or other adults. How to reconcile widely held mental health assumptions with divergent parental cultural values represents an ongoing challenge for clinicians working with diverse families. Some parental child-rearing practices may be misinterpreted by the clinician as indicating severe psychopathology when these practices are not understood in the context of the family's socioeconomic or historical circumstances. Conversely, there is a danger that efforts at cultural sensitivity may unwittingly result in a cultural relativism that overlooks the damage caused to infants/young children by socially sanctioned practices such as harsh punishment, which may have historical roots in the oppression of one cultural group by another but may currently perpetuate a pattern of victimization from the parent to the infant/young child.

The outline in Table 1 presents an approach to incorporating cultural perspectives in the mental health assessment of infants/young children (Sarche, Tsethlikai, Godoy, Emde, & Fleming, in press). It represents an adaptation to the text concerning young children in the DSM–5 Outline for Cultural Formulation (American Psychiatric Association, 2013) and has the goal of helping clinicians reflect on the different facets of cultural identity and their possible influence on the clinical presentation of the infant/young child and the family.

Table 1. Cultural Formulation for Use With Infants and Toddlers

1. Cultural Identity of the Individual

Cultural Identity of Child and Caregivers

Note the ethnic or cultural reference group for the child's parents, and if relevant, other significant caregivers. Cultural reference groups, in addition to race, ethnicity, national origin, and acculturation, may also include gender, gender identity, sexual orientation, religion, socio-economic status.

Note how the parents/caregivers intend to raise the child with respect to their own ethnic or cultural reference group and, in particular, whether or not there are potential issues of multiculturality for the child. For immigrants and ethnic minority families, note the degree of involvement with both the culture of origin and the host culture, and whether or not they anticipate any generational issues with respect to the involvement of the child in the culture of origin and host culture. Note here parent/caregiver language abilities, use, and preference (including multilingualism) and what language(s) they intend to teach the child.

Table 1. Cultural Formulation for Use With Infants and Toddlers (continued)

2. Cultural Conceptualizations of Distress

Cultural Explanations of the Child's Presenting Problem

Note here who first noticed the problem (e.g., parent, other relative, daycare provider, physician) and, if referred by someone else, the extent to which the parents/caregivers also see a problem. Examine whether there is a conflict between parent's awareness and the extended family's awareness of the problem within the context of cultural norms and traditions. Identify what the parents/caregivers observed to be the signals of distress displayed by the infant/toddler (i.e., how did the parents/caregivers know there was a problem); the meaning and perceived severity of the infants distress in relation to the parents'/caregivers' expectations for the behavior and/or development of other infants/toddlers in their community/cultural group; whether there are any local illness categories to describe the child's presenting problem; the parents'/caregivers' perceptions about the cause of, or explanatory models for, the child's presenting problem; and parents'/caregivers' beliefs about treatment of the child's presenting problem (including: previous experiences with dominant and non-dominant culture forms of treatment; current beliefs about and preferences for Western and non-Western forms of treatment; and beliefs about who should be involved in the treatment).

3. Psychosocial Stressors and Cultural Features of Vulnerability and Resilience

Cultural Factors Related to the Child's Psychosocial and Caregiving Environment

A. Infant's Life Space and Environment. Note description of child's physical life space, including community factors (e.g., ethnic/racial composition, urbanicity, crime, and cohesion) and home factors (e.g., people living in the home, their relationship to one another and the child, and presence of extended family and/or others), infant's sleeping arrangements, and parents'/caregivers' culturally relevant interpretations of social supports and stressors (e.g., role of religion, community, and kin networks).

B. Infant's Caregiving Network. Note here the significant caregivers in the child's life, including the role and extent of involvement of primary (e.g., mother, father) and secondary caregivers (e.g., grandparents, siblings, community child care providers, others). Note significant continuities and disruptions in the child's caregiving network (e.g., child's mobility between caregivers and the extent to which this mobility is fluid, predictable, and consistent versus the extent to which this mobility is unpredictable, inconsistent, and/or disrupted) and the extent to which these continuities or disruptions are normative within local culture.

(continued)

(continued)

C. Parents'/Caregivers' Beliefs about Parenting and Child Development. Note here any beliefs about parenting and child development not noted elsewhere, including range of views or discrepancies among parents/caregivers, such as: ceremonial practices (e.g., naming), beliefs about gender roles, disciplinary practices, goals and aspirations for child, belief systems about children and child development, sources parents/caregivers turn to for advice about parenting, beliefs about parenting/caregiving role, etc.

4. Cultural Features of the Relationship Between the Individual and the Clinician

Cultural Elements of the Relationship Between the Parents/ Caregivers and the Clinician

Indicate differences in culture and social status between the child's parents/caregivers and the clinician and any problems these differences may cause in diagnosis and treatment. This may include differences in understanding the child's distress, communication difficulties due to language, communication styles, or understanding about the involvement of others (e.g., extended kin) in the diagnosis and treatment process. Note how parents may perceive the role of the clinician and the parents' level of comfort with help seeking. Also note how the parents'/caregivers' past experience with clinicians or treatment/service systems impacts on the current clinical relationship. These considerations are reflected in the Irving Harris Foundation Professional Development Network's Diversity-Informed Infant Mental Health Tenets (Ghosh Ippen, Noroña, & Thomas, 2012).

5. Overall Cultural Assessment

Overall Cultural Assessment for Child's Diagnosis and Care

Summarize the implications of the components of the cultural formulation identified in earlier sections of the Outline for comprehensive diagnosis and care of the child and support of the parent/caregiver–child relationship.

Note: Table 1 used with permission, Michelle Sarche, Monica Tsethlikai, Leandra Godoy, Robert Emde, and Candace Fleming (2019). *Cultural Perspectives for Assessing Infants and Young Children*. University of Colorado Denver, Anschutz Medical Campus, and Arizona State University, Children's National Health System.

Beyond DC:0–5

The descriptive approach to classification that DC:0–5 embodies has been much criticized. Focusing on behaviors that cluster without any understanding of pathophysiology and etiology is a significant constraint. Also, there is increasing evidence that most forms of psychopathology exist on a continuum, leading to an arbitrariness about defining cut points and "caseness." Categorical disorders involve clustering symptoms that often do not indicate etiology or pathogenesis and do not even necessarily indicate which treatment will be most effective.

DC:0–5 appears at a time of unprecedented progress in neuroscience, genetics, immunology, and cell and molecular biology. These advances bring with them the promise of identifying biomarkers and delineating circuitry involved in the pathophysiology of mental and developmental disorders. Such developments are much needed to increase the precision of diagnoses and treatment and to develop individualized care for infants/young children and their developmental trajectories.

The National Institute of Mental Health in the United States has initiated the Research Domain Criteria (RDoC) project. The RDoC project classifies mental disorders by incorporating multiple dimensions: behavior, thought patterns, neurobiological measures, and genetics. In fact, the RDoC project has changed funding priorities in favor of dimensional approaches.

This does not mean that biological reductionism will hold sway in the future. Evidence is already abundant that environmental and contextual characteristics of individual infants/young children are inextricably linked to their underlying biological characteristics. For example, researchers have demonstrated that experiences lead to molecular changes that increase or decrease gene expression. Understanding pathophysiology will never be enough, but it will likely enhance our effectiveness in relieving suffering and restoring functioning.

Nevertheless, in our view, these developments are not within reach in the intermediate future. Epigenetics is an important research endeavor, but it has no clinical applicability at this time. Even dimensional measures of psychopathology pose challenges for evaluating caseness, which determines whether a clinical condition warrants intervention at the given time. In every clinical encounter, a clinician makes a categorical decision about whether intervention is warranted.

Growing evidence bases ensure that evolution of the diagnostic constructs will continue and that future iterations of the diagnostic classification system will be derived from ongoing and future research. The texts of each disorder in this nosology highlight the evidence on which the criteria were derived and identify the areas of opportunity for future research. At the present state of knowledge, we believe that the descriptive criteria of DC:0–5 are clinically relevant and more useful to practitioners than alternative approaches.

Axis I
Clinical Disorders

10 NEURODEVELOPMENTAL DISORDERS

Neurodevelopmental disorders are a group of disorders with varied manifestations, but they share several common features: an onset in early childhood, a delay or abnormality in functions strongly related to biological maturation of the central nervous system, and a generally steady course that does not involve remissions and relapses that are more typical of other mental disorders. Most neurodevelopmental disorders also are more common in males than females. Genetic factors are implicated in the etiology because family histories of similar or related disorders are common. Research to date suggests that genetic influences are complex—they are not the result of a few specific genetic abnormalities but rather are due to normal variations in multiple genes affected by different environmental conditions. In addition to genetics, environmental neurotoxins (e.g., lead exposure), medical complications (e.g., preterm birth), and social factors (e.g., institutional rearing) also have been implicated as contributors to neurodevelopmental disorders.

The prevalence of these disorders is 15% in industrialized countries. The prevalence in early childhood may be somewhat lower because not all neurodevelopmental disorders are identified in the early childhood years (e.g., specific learning disorders). Different neurodevelopmental disorders co-occur with such high frequency that some researchers have suggested that they may represent different manifestations of a single, overarching disorder. Nevertheless, at this time, there are sufficiently large differences in clinical presentations, correlates, and responses to interventions that justify considering a number of distinct disorders.

Neurodevelopmental disorders are believed to be treatable but not often curable. Early and intensive interventions are recommended for infants/young children with neurodevelopmental disorders. Although these disorders have been linked to brain dysfunction, there is ample evidence that many conditions are improved by psychosocial interventions. Because of the complexity of neurodevelopmental disorders, it is important that multiple disciplines work collaboratively on both assessment and interventions.

In this section, the two best known and best studied neurodevelopmental disorders, Autism Spectrum Disorder (ASD) and Attention Deficit Hyperactivity Disorder (ADHD), are defined. In addition, two disorders that represent early, incomplete manifestations of these disorders (i.e., they include some symptoms and cause impaired functioning) are defined. Early Atypical Autism Spectrum Disorder involves impairing features of ASD but without the full symptom picture. Similarly, Overactivity Disorder of Toddlerhood affects young children who are impaired by symptoms of hyperactivity but do not necessarily meet criteria for ADHD. Each of these disorders derive from longitudinal data in high-risk samples of infants/young children, many of whom eventually manifest full criteria for ASD and for ADHD, respectively.

Three other developmental disorders are also defined: Global Developmental Delay, Developmental Language Disorder, and Developmental Coordination Disorder. These disorders may occur alone, but more often, they occur in combination with other neurodevelopmental disorders. For children with significant developmental delays, clinicians should use the child's mental age in considering Axis I diagnosis.

10.1 Autism Spectrum Disorder

Introduction

Autism Spectrum Disorder (ASD), a neurodevelopmental disorder, is characterized by severe impairments in social interaction and communication and by the presence of restrictive and repetitive behaviors. Accurate and early identification of ASD is critical, particularly given the high prevalence, family and societal costs, and recognized importance of early intervention.

Diagnostic Algorithm

All of the following criteria must be met.

A. Each of the following three social-communication symptoms must be present:

1. Limited or atypical social–emotional responsivity, sustained social attention, or social reciprocity as evidenced by at least one of the following:

   a. Atypical social approach.

   b. Reduced or limited ability to engage in reciprocal social games or activities that require turn-taking (e.g., peek-a-boo).

   c. Reduced or limited ability to initiate joint attention to share interests or emotions or to seek information about objects of interest in the environment.

   d. Infrequent or restricted responses to social interaction.

   e. Rare and restricted, or lack of, initiation of social interaction.

2. Deficits in nonverbal social-communication behaviors as evidenced by at least one of the following:

   a. Lack of or restricted integration of nonverbal and verbal behaviors.

   b. Atypical use of eye contact and turning away from others in social contexts.

    c. Difficulties understanding or using nonverbal communication (e.g., gestures).

    d. Restricted range of facial expressions and limited nonverbal communication.

  3. Peer interaction difficulties as evidenced by at least one of the following:

    a. Problems adapting behavior to accommodate varying social demands across social contexts.

    b. Difficulties engaging in spontaneous pretend or imaginative play.

    c. Limited or lack of interest in peers and in playing with other infants/ young children.

B. Symptoms in criterion A are not better explained by sensory impairment (e.g., vision, hearing, or other major sensory deficit).

C. Two of the following four repetitive and restrictive behaviors must be present:

  1. Stereotyped or repetitive babbling or speech, motor movements, or use of objects and toys.

  2. Rigidly maintains routines with excessive resistance to change; demands sameness and shows distress in response to change or transitions; or ritualized use of stereotyped, odd, or idiosyncratic verbal phrases, or nonverbal behaviors.

  3. Highly circumscribed, specific, or unusual interests that manifest in extreme or atypical fixation on an item or topic of interest.

  4. Atypical responsivity to sensory inputs (either over- or under-responsive) or unusual engagement with sensory aspects of the environment (e.g., licking carpet).

D. Symptoms of the disorder, or caregiver accommodations in response to the symptoms, significantly affect the infant's/young child's and family's functioning in one or more of the following ways:

  1. Cause distress to the infant/young child;

  2. Interfere with the infant's/young child's relationships;

  3. Limit the infant's/young child's participation in developmentally expected activities or routines;

  4. Limit the family's participation in everyday activities or routines; or

  5. Limit the infant's/young child's ability to learn and develop new skills or interfere with developmental progress.

Age: The diagnosis should be made with caution in young children less than 18 months old.

Duration: There are no duration criteria for the presence of symptoms.

Specify:

1. With or without Global Developmental Delay

2. With or without language delay

3. Associated with a known genetic condition or environmental factor

4. Associated with sensory processing abnormalities

Note: Infants/young children who show unexplained regression or abrupt increase in restrictive and repetitive behaviors should receive a comprehensive medical evaluation. Infants/young children less than 30 months old for whom there are marked concerns in social development, but whose symptoms do not meet criteria for ASD, should be evaluated for Early Atypical Autism Spectrum Disorder.

Diagnostic Features

The symptom criteria that are used to diagnose ASD in infants/young children are the same as those used to diagnose ASD in older children, adolescents, and adults. However, the specific behavioral manifestations of the social-communication symptoms are different because infants/young children have more limited social-communication and interpersonal-relationship skills. For example, infants/young children are not expected to ask other infants/young children or adults about their experiences or to be able to reflect on their own emotional experiences.

Associated Features Supporting Diagnosis

Many infants/young children who go on to receive a diagnosis of ASD come to the attention of clinicians because the parents are concerned about the infant/young child being delayed in language and communication. Indeed, many infants/young children with ASD have significant expressive and receptive language delays at the time of diagnosis. Global Developmental Delay is also common. Several additional risk factors increase the likelihood of an ASD diagnosis. The most compelling is when an infant/young child is a younger sibling of a child who is diagnosed with ASD, as the risk appears to be approximately 19%, with higher risk for boys and for infants/young children who have more than one older sibling with an ASD diagnosis. In addition, there is evidence that infants who are born preterm are at higher risk for developing ASD.

Developmental Features

There is wide individual variation in developmental trajectories of infants/young children who develop ASD. Both social-communication and repetitive and restricted behaviors may appear in the first year of life. Age at onset varies between 12 and 36 months old. There is marked variation in the emergence of a spectrum of social and communicative deficits. Some young children evidence marked loss or regression in social-communication and language skills, whereas others show a more gradual pattern of onset, which may be marked by failure to acquire age-appropriate social skills or a gradual disengagement from social interaction. Most parents report developmental concern between

18 and 24 months old. However, infants/young children without developmental delays tend to be diagnosed at later ages, in preschool or later as the demands of social interaction increase. Many infants/young children with ASD and global or language delays show marked gains in language and cognitive development throughout early childhood.

Prevalence

Once considered rare, ASD is now among the most common neurodevelopmental disorders, with current estimates in the United States at 1 in 68 children. Given that boys are approximately 4 times more likely to be affected than girls, the estimated prevalence for boys is 1 in 42, and for girls it is 1 in 189.

Course

ASD diagnoses made prior to 3 years old have been found to be significantly stable over time, although stability increases when diagnoses are made after 4 years old.

Risk and Prognostic Features

Several factors have been associated with increased risk for ASD, including having an older sibling with ASD or other familial/genetic risk; being male; having a global developmental delay, intellectual disability, or language delay; being born preterm or with low birthweight; having older parents; and being exposed to environmental toxins (e.g., prenatal exposure to valproate, proximity to a highway). In addition, some genetic conditions, such as Fragile X syndrome and Tuberous Sclerosis Complex, are associated with elevated risk for ASD. Some studies have found that children with higher language and cognitive functioning and those with relatively enhanced joint attention skills attain more positive outcomes.

Culture-Related Diagnostic Issues

There are known health disparities in age at diagnosis and rates of diagnosis in the United States. Infants/young children with ASD who are raised in poverty, raised by parents who are not native English speakers, or who are raised by parents who identify as racial/ethnic minorities have historically been diagnosed at later ages or are misdiagnosed as having only an intellectual disability. As there are cultural variations in social-communication practices and emotion expression, an infant's/young child's symptoms must be evaluated in the context of his or her family's and community's cultural practices.

Gender-Related Diagnostic Issues

Although the prevalence of ASD has gone up dramatically, the ratio of affected boys to girls has remained stable, with boys being approximately 3–4 times more likely to receive a diagnosis of ASD.

Differential Diagnosis

Infants/young children with Rett syndrome may present with ASD symptoms in early childhood. When an intellectual disability or Global Developmental Delay is very severe, it can be challenging to distinguish ASD from Global Developmental Delay. It is important to evaluate social-communication symptoms in the context of the infant's/young child's mental age—particularly when examining social deficits. Infants/young children with Reactive Attachment Disorder may show impairments in social reciprocity and Global Developmental Delays, but they should show selective absence of attachment behaviors, language delays comparable with cognitive delays, and no evidence of repetitive and restricted behaviors other than motor stereotypies.

Comorbidity

Global Developmental Delay and language delays are very common among infants/young children with ASD. Formal developmental assessment is important for characterizing the infant's/young child's functioning, with the recognition that both language and cognitive scores are less stable in early childhood. Infants/young children with ASD often show uneven cognitive profiles. Furthermore, it is not unusual for young children with ASD to evidence higher expressive than receptive language skills (e.g., functional, scripted two-word utterances and counting skills with limited language understanding). Deficits in social communication affect day-to-day adaptive functioning; discrepancies between cognitive and adaptive functioning are common. In addition to repetitive motor movements (e.g., toe-walking, posturing, flapping), infants/young children with ASD may evidence motor delays/deficits, such as clumsiness or unusual gait. Some infants/young children with ASD may evidence significant hyperactivity or inattention to both social and nonsocial stimuli. In these instances, it is appropriate to consider a diagnosis of Attention Deficit Hyperactivity Disorder. Older children with ASD exhibit elevated rates of anxiety and depression. Finally, infants/young children with ASD display high rates of challenging behaviors, including sleep and eating problems, negative emotionality, and self-injurious behaviors.

Links to DSM–5 and ICD–10

DSM–5: Autism Spectrum Disorder
ICD–10: Childhood Autism (F84.0)

10.2 Early Atypical Autism Spectrum Disorder

Introduction

Early Atypical Autism Spectrum Disorder (EAASD) characterizes severe social-communication abnormalities and restricted and repetitive symptoms in infants/young children between 9 and 36 months old who have not ever met full criteria for Autism Spectrum Disorder (ASD). The diagnostic threshold for EAASD requires two of the three social-communication symptoms and one of the four restrictive and repetitive symptoms.

Inclusion of EAASD in the DC:0–5™ is informed by current understanding of ASD symptom progression that has emerged from studies of infant siblings of children with ASD. A consistent pattern of findings reveals a broad window of risk for the emergence of full ASD criteria, marked by variability in age at onsets for relatively stable ASD diagnoses that occur between 12 and 36 months as well as patterns of slow regression through the window of risk for many infants/young children who go on to meet full DSM–5 criteria for ASD. The EAASD diagnosis identifies infants/young children with serious, persistent, and impairing ASD symptomatology who are subthreshold for ASD.

EAASD applies only to infants/young children who are between 9 and 36 months old and who have impaired functioning from their symptomatology but who do not have sufficient numbers of symptoms to meet full DSM–5 ASD diagnostic criteria. This diagnosis is not intended to apply to infants/young children whose behavior is better explained by a language or intellectual delay/disability/disorder or other psychopathology. Infants/young children with EAASD are believed to be at high risk for developing ASD and should be monitored for the development of new symptoms.

Diagnostic Algorithm

At least two social-communication criteria and one repetitive and restrictive behavior criterion must be met, as well as the impairment criterion.

A. Two of the following three social-communication symptoms must be present:

1. Limited or atypical social–emotional responsivity, sustained social attention, or social reciprocity as evidenced by at least one of the following:

   a. Atypical social approach.

   b. Reduced or limited ability to engage in reciprocal social games or activities that require turn-taking (e.g., peek-a-boo).

   c. Reduced or limited ability to initiate joint attention to shared interests or emotions or to seek information about objects of interest in the environment.

   d. Infrequent or restricted responses to social interaction or rare, restricted, and lack of initiation of social interaction.

   e. Rare and restricted, or lack of, initiation of social interaction.

2. Deficits in nonverbal social-communication behaviors as evidenced by at least one of the following:

   a. Lack of or restricted integration of nonverbal and verbal behaviors.

   b. Atypical use of eye contact and turning away from others in social contexts.

    c. Difficulties understanding or using nonverbal communication (e.g., gestures).

    d. Restricted range of facial expressions and limited nonverbal communication.

3. Peer interaction difficulties as evidenced by at least one of the following:

    a. Problems adapting behavior to accommodate varying social demands across social contexts.

    b. Difficulties engaging in spontaneous pretend or imaginative play.

    c. Limited or lack of interest in peers and in playing with other infants/young children.

B. Symptoms in criterion A are not better explained by sensory impairment (e.g., vision, hearing, or other major sensory deficit). The infant/young child does not meet criteria for ASD.

C. One of the following four repetitive and restrictive behaviors must be present:

1. Stereotyped or repetitive babbling or speech, motor movements, or use of objects and toys.

2. Rigidly maintains routines with excessive resistance to change; demands sameness and shows distress in response to change or transitions; or ritualized use of stereotyped, odd, or idiosyncratic verbal phrases, or nonverbal behaviors.

3. Highly circumscribed, specific, or unusual interests that manifest in extreme or atypical fixation on an item or topic of interest.

4. Atypical responsivity to sensory inputs (either over- or under-responsive) or unusual engagement with sensory aspects of the environment (e.g., licking carpet).

D. Symptoms of the disorder, or caregiver accommodations in response to the symptoms, significantly affect the infant's/young child's and family's functioning in one or more of the following ways:

1. Cause distress to the infant/young child;

2. Interfere with the infant's/young child's relationships;

3. Limit the infant's/young child's participation in developmentally expected activities or routines;

4. Limit the family's participation in everyday activities or routines; or

5. Limit the infant's/young child's ability to learn and develop new skills or interfere with developmental progress.

Age: The diagnosis of EAASD can only be made between 9 and 36 months old. Preschool-age children who meet criteria for EAASD should be evaluated for the DSM–5 Social (Pragmatic) Communication Disorder.

Duration: There are no duration criteria for the presence of symptoms.

Specify:

1. With or without Global Developmental Delay

2. With or without language delay

3. Associated with a known genetic condition or environmental factor

4. Associated with sensory processing abnormalities

Note: Infants/young children who show unexplained regression or abrupt increase in restrictive and repetitive behaviors should receive a comprehensive medical evaluation.

Diagnostic Features

The symptom criteria that are used to diagnose EAASD in infants/young children are the same as those used to diagnose ASD in older children, adolescents, and adults. However, the specific behavioral manifestations of the social-communication symptoms are different because infants/young children have more limited social-communication and interpersonal-relationship skills. For example, infants/young children are not expected to ask other infants/young children or adults about their experiences or to be able to reflect on their own emotional experiences.

Associated Features Supporting Diagnosis

Consistent with ASD, many infants/young children who receive a diagnosis of EAASD may come to the attention of clinicians because their caregivers are concerned about the infant/young child being delayed in language and communication. Assuming that some infants/young children diagnosed with EAASD are showing early symptoms of ASD as part of the progression of ASD, and given that many infants/young children with ASD have significant expressive and receptive language delays as well as Global Developmental Delays at the time of diagnosis, it is important to evaluate infants'/young children's expressive, receptive, and cognitive functioning.

Developmental Features

Although data for EAASD are not available, on the basis of findings about the progression of ASD, it is likely that there will be individual variation in developmental trajectories of infants/young children who develop EAASD. Both social-communication and repetitive and restricted behaviors may appear in the first year of life. Age at onset varies, although some symptoms may be present in the first year of life. There is marked variation in the emergence of a spectrum of social and communicative deficits. Some young children exhibit marked loss or regression in social-communication and language skills, whereas others show a more gradual pattern of onset, which may be marked by failure to acquire age-appropriate social skills or a gradual disengagement from social interaction. Infants/young children who meet criteria for EAASD should be monitored for the emergence of additional symptoms because they are at very high risk for developing ASD.

Prevalence

The prevalence of EAASD is unknown, but the prevalence of ASD appears to have increased in recent years.

Course

The course of EAASD is unknown. Infants as young as 12 months who manifest multiple social-communicative and restricted/repetitive symptoms are at increased risk for developing ASD, but the course of EAASD has not been delineated.

Risk and Prognostic Features

It is likely that the same risk factors that have been associated with ASD—including having an older sibling with ASD or other familial/genetic risk; being male; having Global Developmental Delay, intellectual disability, or language delay; being born preterm or with low birthweight; having older parents; and being exposed to environmental toxins (e.g., prenatal exposure to valproate, proximity to a highway)—are associated with the onset of EAASD. There is evidence that infants/young children who develop full ASD symptoms prior to 2 years old and those who develop symptoms at or after 2 years old are indistinguishable by 3 years old in terms of the severity of symptoms. There is also emerging evidence that treating infants/young children who have ASD symptoms, whether they meet full ASD criteria, can minimize social-communication deficits.

Culture-Related Diagnostic Issues

There are cultural variations in social-communication practices and emotion expression. Therefore, an infant's/young child's symptoms must be evaluated in the context of his or her family's and community's cultural practices.

Gender-Related Diagnostic Issues

There are no data on gender differences for EAASD. However, there is evidence that boys are more likely to show elevated risk on questionnaires and observational ASD screeners, even prior to the ages at which infants/young children typically receive ASD diagnoses (i.e., 12 months old).

Differential Diagnosis

Infants/young children with Rett syndrome may present with ASD symptoms in early childhood. When an intellectual disability or Global Developmental Delay is very severe, it can be challenging to distinguish EAASD and ASD symptoms from Global Developmental Delay. It is important to evaluate social-communication symptoms in the context of the infant's/young child's mental age—particularly when examining social deficits. Infants/young children with Reactive Attachment Disorder may show impairments in social reciprocity and Global Developmental Delays, but they should show selective absence of attachment behaviors, language delays comparable with cognitive delays, and no evidence of repetitive and restricted behaviors other than motor stereotypies.

Comorbidity

There are no data on comorbidity for EAASD. However, ASD symptoms are elevated among infants/young children with Global Developmental Delay and language delays. Formal developmental assessment is important for characterizing the infant's/young child's functioning, with the recognition that both language and cognitive scores are less stable in early childhood.

Links to DSM–5 and ICD–10

DSM–5: Other Specified Neurodevelopmental Disorder
ICD–10: Pervasive Developmental Disorder, Unspecified (F84.9)

10.3 Attention Deficit Hyperactivity Disorder

Introduction

Attention Deficit Hyperactivity Disorder (ADHD) is a disorder of developmentally inappropriate levels of inattention or hyperactivity–impulsivity that interfere with the functioning of a young child and his or her family. Although young children have higher levels of inattention, hyperactivity, and impulsivity than older children, some young children present with extremes of these patterns even at early ages, allowing for identification of those young children with specific difficulties in these areas.

Symptoms of ADHD are among the most common reasons for referral to mental health professionals in early childhood. Given the potential differential diagnosis that includes typical development as well as many other mental health diagnoses, rigorous application of the diagnosis is necessary. Young children with symptoms in only one context or only one relationship should not be diagnosed with ADHD, and young children who have fewer symptoms than required also should not receive this diagnosis. Conversely, young children who meet the criteria should be diagnosed with the disorder to ensure access to appropriate support and treatment and to facilitate effective communication across providers.

Diagnostic Algorithm

All of the following criteria must be met.

A. Present with at least six symptoms from the inattention cluster or at least six symptoms from the hyperactivity–impulsivity cluster.

   1. Inattention Cluster

      a. Usually is not careful and is inattentive to details in play, activities of daily living, or structured activities (e.g., makes developmentally unexpected accidents or mistakes).

      b. Usually has a hard time maintaining focus on activities or play.

c. Often fails to attend to verbal requests/demands, especially when engaged in a preferred activity (e.g., caregiver needs to call the young child's name multiple times before he or she appears to notice).

d. Often gets derailed when attempting to follow multistep instructions and does not complete the activity.

e. Often has a hard time executing age-appropriate sequential activities (e.g., getting dressed, following routines in child care or home).

f. Frequently avoids or objects to activities that require prolonged attention (e.g., reading a book with a parent or working on a puzzle).

g. Loses track of things that are used regularly (e.g., favorite stuffed animal, shoes, or a school bag).

h. Frequently gets distracted by sounds and sights (e.g., sounds from another room or objects or activities out the window).

i. Frequently seems to forget what he or she is doing in common routines or activities.

2. Hyperactivity–Impulsivity Cluster

a. Frequently squirms or fidgets when expected to be still, even for short periods of time.

b. Usually gets up from seat during activities when sitting is expected (e.g., circle time, mealtime, worship).

c. Often climbs on furniture or other inappropriate objects.

d. Usually seems to make more noise than other young children and has difficulty playing quietly.

e. Often shows excessive motor activity and nondirected energy (as if "driven by a motor").

f. Usually talks too much.

g. Often has a hard time taking turns in conversation or interrupts others in conversations (e.g., talks over others).

h. Often has difficulty taking turns in activities or waiting for needs to be met.

i. Is frequently intrusive in play or other activities (e.g., takes over toys or activities from other young children, interrupts an established game).

B. Symptoms in criterion A must be excessive when compared with developmentally and culturally expected norms.

C. Symptoms must be confirmed to be present in at least two contexts of the young child's life (e.g., two different physical settings [home and out-of-home settings] or within two different relationships [caregiver, teacher/child care provider, clinician]).

D. Symptoms of the disorder, or caregiver accommodations in response to the symptoms, significantly affect the young child's and family's functioning in one or more of the following ways:

1. Cause distress to the young child;

2. Cause distress to family;

3. Interfere with the young child's relationships;

4. Limit the young child's participation in developmentally expected activities or routines;

5. Limit the family's participation in everyday activities or routines; or

6. Limit the young child's ability to learn and develop new skills or interfere with developmental progress.

Age: The young child must be at least 36 months old.

Duration: The symptoms must be present for at least 6 months.

Diagnostic Features

Overactivity and impulsivity, coupled with inattentiveness, are core features of this disorder. These behavioral patterns are more pervasive and more extreme than is typical for same-age peers and are evident in at least two settings. A necessary feature for an ADHD diagnosis is the presence of functional impairment. Functional consequences of ADHD typically include difficult relationships among the young child and caregivers, peers, and teachers. Other documented consequences include physical injury, risky behavior, disruptions of class, and difficulties with peers.

Associated Features Supporting Diagnosis

Young children with ADHD in the preschool years are at higher risk of other developmental delays, including mild intellectual impairment, developmental deficits, poor preacademic skills, motor coordination problems, and difficulties in social interactions. Preschoolers with ADHD also have executive functioning deficits. They may receive special education services (or be eligible for these supports) at higher rates than typically developing young children.

School suspensions and expulsions are not uncommon in young children with the disorder and can lead to financial hardships for parents as well as psychological consequences in the young child. In addition, some of the most prevalent difficulties linked to ADHD are learning problems and academic failure.

Not all young children with ADHD will have a family history of attention problems or hyperactivity–impulsivity. However, the presence of a family history of ADHD is an important associated feature for young children who meet criteria for ADHD.

Developmental Features

Hyperactivity and impulsivity are stable constructs over time beginning in toddlerhood. Compared with school-age children, preschoolers are more likely to present with symptoms from the hyperactivity–impulsivity cluster, with about one quarter of children meeting criteria for this pattern, compared with very few 12-year-olds. The stability of these diagnoses based on the domain of symptoms (i.e., inattention or hyperactivity–impulsivity), however, is limited, and young children commonly switch between symptom domains with age. For young children less than 24 months old, Overactivity Disorder of Toddlerhood should be considered.

Prevalence

In young children 2–6 years old, most studies report prevalence rates in the 2%–6% range, although rates from 0.4% to 8.8% have been reported in some samples.

Course

The predictive validity of hyperactivity and impulsivity at 18 months predicting an ADHD diagnosis at 36 months is modest, although statistically significant. The symptom clusters of hyperactivity, impulsivity, and inattention are inconsistent over time. ADHD in young children, however, is relatively persistent across time. Stability of signs of ADHD increase as children become older. Therefore, stability in preschoolers is greater than in toddlers, but less than in school age children. Young children with ADHD are at much higher risk for learning disorders and academic problems in the school-age period. ADHD symptoms in young children are predictive of depression in young adulthood as well as later conduct disorders.

Risk and Prognostic Features

Genetic and environmental factors, including abuse and neglect, have been linked to increased risk for ADHD in early childhood. For example, young children raised in adverse caregiving environments, such as institutions or orphanages, have approximately a fourfold risk of ADHD in early childhood compared with nonmaltreated preschoolers living in families. Specific caregiving patterns, such as intrusive caregiving, are especially associated with inattentiveness and hyperactivity. Heritability of hyperactivity in young children is approximately 70%, similar to rates in older children. Research into the specific genes related to ADHD has occurred primarily in older children. Attention has focused on genes related to dopaminergic and other catecholamine activity and metabolism. As with most disorders, it is most likely that ADHD in young children develops in the context of complex interactions among genetic and environmental factors. Specific neurodevelopmental syndromes, including Fragile X syndrome and Autism Spectrum Disorder, are associated with high rates of ADHD.

Noninherited prenatal and postnatal factors are also associated with signs of preschool ADHD. Prenatal exposure to maternal substance abuse, including alcohol use, is associated with signs of preschool ADHD. Findings related to the association between preschool ADHD and prenatal smoking exposure are mixed, with many, but not all, studies reporting an association. Perinatal factors, including low birthweight and preterm birth, also predict early hyperactivity and impulsivity. Postnatal exposure to lead and central nervous system disorders, such as seizures, are also associated with higher rates of ADHD. Family factors—including young parental age, parental depression, and having an isolated family—also increase risk of preschool ADHD.

Culture-Related Diagnostic Issues

Rates of ADHD symptoms in early childhood appear similar across cultures. The modest variability in rates of diagnosis—that is, the individual criteria plus impairment—suggests that cultural expectations about developmentally appropriate behaviors may affect the meaning of functional impairment, which is required for the diagnosis.

Gender-Related Diagnostic Issues

Some studies of young children indicate that boys have a greater prevalence of ADHD than girls, although the magnitude of this difference is somewhat less than in older children.

Differential Diagnosis

For all young children, clinicians must consider the differential diagnosis of typical development, a relationship disorder, Posttraumatic Stress Disorder, or other Axis I disorder before making a diagnosis of ADHD. Typical development may include a high level of symptoms but generally does not cause substantial impairment. Difficulty meeting inappropriate developmental expectations, such as a requirement for young children to sit alone at a desk doing "school work" for extended periods of time, does not constitute functional impairment. Relationship disorders may present with relationship-specific symptoms or distorted perceptions about a young child's presentation. Posttraumatic Stress Disorder may cause hyperarousal symptoms and distress that present as disorganized behaviors, but signs of Posttraumatic Stress Disorder should be linked to exposure or reminders to the potentially traumatic event. Sleep disorders that cause sleep deprivation, including sleep apnea, can present with behavioral patterns similar to ADHD. Many other disorders—including other anxiety disorders and mood disorders—may cause behavioral dysregulation, but ADHD does not include a pervasive mood or anxiety pattern. Lead toxicity should be considered as an etiologic factor in young children with signs of ADHD. Absence seizures may present with signs that are suggestive of inattention symptoms, but they may be distinguished because young children with a seizure will not respond to verbal cues during the brief epileptic events.

Comorbidity

ADHD frequently co-occurs with other psychiatric disorders, with a large majority of preschool-age children with ADHD meeting diagnostic criteria for other disorders. Specific patterns of comorbidity vary across the literature, but ADHD can be associated with Oppositional Defiant Disorder, internalizing disorders (specifically, Separation Anxiety Disorder), and Major Depressive Disorder, or with a cluster of Oppositional Defiant Disorder, Major Depressive Disorder, and Generalized Anxiety Disorder.

Links to DSM–5 and ICD–10

DSM–5: Attention Deficit Hyperactivity Disorder
ICD–10: Disturbance of Activity and Attention (F90.1)

10.4 Overactivity Disorder of Toddlerhood

Introduction

Overactivity Disorder of Toddlerhood (OADT) describes a syndrome of pervasive, persistent, extreme, developmentally inappropriate hyperactivity and impulsivity in young children. Although as a group, typically developing young children have higher levels of motor activity and less impulse control than older children, a small proportion of young children present with even higher levels of activity that are sustained and predictive of high levels of activity through the school-age years. Hyperactivity alone does not constitute a clinical syndrome. Young children with the clinical syndrome of OADT must have high activity and experience impairment, such as exclusion from activities, problems in relationships with others, or concerns about safe behavior. The disorder derives its validity primarily from studies using continuous measures of activity rather than categorical measures, but these studies make clear the importance of early identification for the small percentage of young children who are experiencing extreme symptoms and functional impairment.

Diagnostic Algorithm

All of the following criteria must be met.

A. The young child presents with at least six symptoms from the following that are excessive when compared with developmentally and culturally expected norms:

1. Frequently squirms or fidgets when expected to be still, even for short periods of time.

2. Usually gets up or attempts to get up from seat during activities when sitting is expected (e.g., circle time, mealtime, car seat).

3. Often climbs on furniture or other inappropriate objects.

4. Usually seems to make more noise than other young children and has difficulty playing quietly.

5. Often shows excessive motor activity and nondirected energy (as if "driven by a motor").

6. Usually talks too much.

7. Often has a hard time taking turns in conversation or excessively interrupts others in conversations.

8. Often has difficulty taking turns in activities or waiting for needs to be met.

9. Is frequently intrusive in play, interactions, or other activities (e.g., takes over toys or activities from other young children, interrupts an established game).

B. Behaviors meeting the criteria below must be excessive when compared with developmentally and culturally expected norms.

C. Symptoms must be confirmed to be present in at least two contexts of the young child's life (e.g., two different physical settings [home and out-of-home settings] or within two different relationships [caregiver, teacher or child care provider, clinician]).

D. Symptoms of the disorder, or caregiver accommodations in response to the symptoms, significantly affect the young child's and family's functioning in one or more of the following ways:

1. Cause distress to the young child;

2. Interfere with the young child's relationships;

3. Limit the young child's participation in developmentally expected activities or routines;

4. Limit the family's participation in everyday activities or routines; or

5. Limit the young child's ability to learn and develop new skills or interfere with developmental progress.

Age: The young child is older than 24 months and younger than 36 months.

Duration: The symptoms must be present for at least 6 months.

Diagnostic Features

The disorder derives from consistent identification of young children exhibiting hyperactivity and impulsivity with impaired functioning. These behaviors have a well-described neurodevelopmental trajectory that may begin during toddlerhood. Early identification is particularly important for young children for whom family-focused interventions may be effective in symptom reduction and may positively influence the developmental trajectory.

The developmental window for this disorder is intentionally narrow, with a lower limit of 24 months old, which is the lowest age at which these symptoms have been studied as a categorical diagnosis, and an upper limit of 36 months old, after which the diagnosis of Attention Deficit Hyperactivity Disorder (ADHD) should be considered.

Activity level is one of the most observable behavioral manifestations of a range of internal experiences of young children, and no etiology is required or specified. As with all disorders, a careful assessment yielding a complete formulation will put this clinical construct into the young child's individual context. An important developmental feature of infancy and early childhood is the reliance on the caregiver for safety and for supporting a young child's behavioral regulation skills. OADT is not a diagnosis focused on the parent's role in this developing process. The diagnosis does not apply when a caregiver perceives a young child as more active than typically developing young children in the context of limited parental structure or oversight but this perception is not supported by a full assessment involving observations and collateral information.

The diagnosis should not be considered in young children with episodic, reactive, or context-specific changes in activity level. In that case, a broad differential diagnosis should be considered, and it is likely that co-occurring disorders also may be present.

Associated Features Supporting Diagnosis

Young children presenting with signs of OADT may have experienced injuries, such as lacerations requiring stitches or head injuries due to falls, related to impulsivity or overactivity. Primary caregivers may report difficulty finding other adults—such as babysitters, extended family, or child care settings—willing to care for the young child. Recent data suggest that early hyperactivity is associated with short sleep duration, a pattern seen commonly in clinical practice, although the direction of causality is not yet established. In addition, physical aggression is often associated with overactivity in young children.

Developmental Features

Data examining the trajectory of overactivity and impulsivity in young children suggest that the level of overactivity is likely to be stable across the short time period that OADT may be diagnosed and is likely to remain stable through the preschool period. Criterion A must be considered in the context of culturally and developmentally appropriate expectations. If a young child is developmentally younger than his or her chronological age and would not be expected to have mastered some of the activities described in criterion A, those criteria should not be used to support the diagnosis.

Criteria A1 and A2 are not intended to apply to prolonged sitting, such as for a full worship service, but to brief periods of time with other people, such as looking at a book, exploring a new toy, or singing a song with a group. For criterion A3, the frequency of the climbing is important to distinguish typical exploration from excessive climbing. Young children with OADT are likely to climb any object, including high or potentially dangerous furniture or structures. Criterion A4 distinguishes the young child's volume explicitly from that of other young children and can be identified in group play as well as solitary play. Criterion A7 describes a symptom in which a parent is unable to have adult conversations without interruption, or other young children cannot play even for brief periods of time without intrusion by the identified young child.

Prevalence

There are limited data examining the rates of the categorical diagnosis of OADT. However, epidemiologic data from Europe and North America demonstrate that 7%–16% of young children show a developmental trajectory of stable, high levels of hyperactivity and impulsivity, not accounting for multisetting and impairment criteria. On the basis of existing data in older children, it is likely that no more than half of young children with hyperactivity and impulsivity might have impairment; however, given the context-specificity of impairment and the different expectations for young children, it is likely that even fewer would meet criteria for OADT.

Course

Epidemiologic data demonstrate high stability in levels of activity over development from toddlerhood during the toddler and early childhood period with modest stability through the school-age period. In studies not examining impairment, a small group of young children show extreme and high levels of hyperactivity and impulsivity over time, with a reduction of hyperactivity and impulsivity for most young children from toddlerhood to school age. The outcomes of the categorical diagnosis have not yet been established, but it is expected that OADT will show substantial continuity with ADHD in the early childhood period.

Risk and Prognostic Features

Persistent overactivity in toddlerhood is associated with a range of biological, relationship, and environmental factors. Biological perinatal factors, including preterm birth and low birthweight, are associated with a twofold risk of persistent and extreme overactivity, as is prenatal nicotine exposure. Family factors—including single parent at birth, low maternal age, food insecurity, maternal depression, and paternal history of antisocial behaviors—have all been found to predict stable hyperactivity behaviors in young children. For young children for whom OADT predicts later ADHD, preschool ADHD risk factors—including genetic factors, hereditable patterns, and caregiving adversity—may also confer risk in toddlerhood.

Culture-Related Diagnostic Issues

Cultural expectations are critically important in defining behavioral expectations and impairment. Although every culture has its own customs and expectations regarding young children's behaviors, cultural norms, by definition, are achievable by most young children in that culture. Thus, the construct of extreme and problematic overactivity is one that could be applied only to the small minority of young children who do not meet that norm. Conversely, if a behavior described in criterion A is not thought to be developmentally expected within a cultural context (e.g., sitting in a chair even for a short time), the presence of those criteria should not be used to support the diagnosis.

As cultural expectations shift, it is important to monitor the number of young children identified as impaired by overactivity to ensure that the expectations continue to be achievable. Studies in North America and Europe demonstrate in older children that the youngest children in the class have substantially higher risk of having been diagnosed with ADHD, suggesting that the culturally sanctioned expectation may not fit the developmental capacity. It is particularly important, therefore, that a similar pattern be avoided in the toddler period and that the diagnosis of OADT only be applied when impairment is assessed in the context of developmentally appropriate expectations, even if culturally sanctioned policies promote developmentally inappropriate expectations.

Gender-Related Diagnostic Issues

In epidemiologic studies, boys fall into the "high" hyperactivity–impulsivity group at twice the rate of girls. Again, culturally related norms must be considered, and clinical caution is warranted if similar severity of symptoms in girls and boys result in different levels of impairment.

Differential Diagnosis

The differential diagnosis for OADT is broad and includes typical development, a relationship-specific disorder, mood or anxiety problems, trauma-related disorders, developmental delay, and sensory or medical issues. Typical development must be considered with any chief complaint of overactivity. Typical development in toddlerhood includes a high level of activity and may cause some challenges to parents' activities of daily living (e.g., grocery shopping), but it does not cause true impairment in the young child's or family's functioning.

Relationship disorders may present with relationship-specific overactivity or distorted perceptions and attributions about a young child's presentation. Mood and anxiety can present with behavioral dysregulation in young children. Early dysregulation related to stressors may present with overactivity but would generally be seen as context-specific or episodic. Young children with developmental delays will often demonstrate levels of activity consistent with their developmental level, which may be more active than expected for their chronological age. OADT should be distinguished from sensory over-reactivity by the context of the overactivity, which is pervasive in OADT but is linked to sensory exposures in Sensory Over-Responsivity Disorder. Sleep deprivation from sleep disorders or environmental factors can present with disturbed behavioral regulation including overactivity but also usually sleep-cycle patterns of sleepiness. Medical conditions may be related to behavioral dysregulation but usually with evidence of pain, growth disturbances, or other physical symptoms. The exception to this rule is lead exposure, which may be silent or present with overactivity and should be considered in all young children with overactivity, especially those with comorbid pica. Some medications—such as steroids, diphenhydramine, and even albuterol absorbed systemically—may be associated with overactivity in young children and should be considered as part of the differential diagnosis.

Comorbidity

Many of the disorders listed previously in the differential diagnosis may also show comorbidity with overactivity. Sleep problems and dysregulated behaviors, such as those seen in Disorder of Dysregulated Anger and Aggression of Early Childhood, are well documented. Because of the association with adversity, trauma-related disorders—such as Posttraumatic Stress Disorder—may also occur comorbidly with OADT when a young child presents with overactivity as well as the signs of Posttraumatic Stress Disorder.

DSM–5: Attention Deficit Hyperactivity Disorder, predominantly hyperactive–impulsive presentation
ICD–10: Disturbance of Activity and Attention (F90.1)

10.5 Global Developmental Delay

Introduction

Global Developmental Delay (GDD) is diagnosed when infants/young children have significantly below average functioning (i.e., delays or deficits) across developmental domains, including verbal and nonverbal reasoning, problem solving, language development, social development, fine and gross motor skills, and adaptive behaviors. GDD is diagnosed instead of intellectual disability in infancy and early childhood to reflect the greater plasticity of early development and the possibility of cognitive and adaptive growth. Similarly, because of the greater plasticity and variability of expectations for infants/young children, severity specifiers based on the degree of adaptive deficits are not included.

The infant/young child shows a consistent pattern of delay across developmental domains on standardized measures of development. Infants/young children with GDD typically have scores that are 1.5–2 or more standard deviations below the mean for their age and cultural group.

The etiology of GDD varies from social neglect to a genetic condition (e.g., Fragile X syndrome, Down syndrome). When GDD occurs in the context of a genetic condition, it is important to determine whether the specific phenotype associated with the genetic condition influences the course of cognitive development because some conditions (e.g., Rett syndrome) may be associated with declining cognitive functioning or a plateau in cognitive functioning.

Although standardized, norm-referenced developmental tests in infancy and the early preschool period are less stable than standardized, norm-referenced IQ tests designed for young children 3–5 years old and older children, adolescents, and adults, many infants/young children with GDD will go on to meet criteria for intellectual disability.

Parents often become aware of their infant's/young child's GDD when he or she does not attain motor milestones (e.g., sitting up, walking) or fails to talk. When any developmental domain is delayed, it is important to pursue formal standardized multidomain assessment. When an infant's/young child's developmental test scores support a GDD diagnosis, it is important to administer a test of adaptive functioning to determine whether the infant's/young child's test performance is supported by his or her everyday performance of skills required for age-appropriate independent functioning.

Infants/young children with GDD usually show patterns of relative strength and weakness across developmental domains that can inform intervention efforts. However, infants/young children with GDD show marked delays in most developmental domains, in contrast to infants/young children with specific learning or language disorders. GDD is associated with a broad range of mental health disorders.

Diagnostic Algorithm

All of the following criteria must be met.

A. Deficits in cognitive functioning, verbal and nonverbal problem solving, planning, symbolic reasoning, motor skills, social judgment, and learning, including preacademic skills in the preschool period, which is confirmed by standardized developmental or intellectual assessment with a norm-referenced assessment tool. These deficits are documented by a delay that is 2 standard deviations below the mean on a test of developmental/intellectual functioning (or within the standard error of 2 standard deviations below the mean; e.g., a standard score less than 75).

B. Deficits in adaptive behavior, which refers to the performance of age-expected communication, social, and daily living skills required for independent day-to-day adaptive functioning. Without supports, the adaptive deficits limit the infant's/young child's participation and engagement in one or more age-expected activities of daily life, such as home routines (e.g., self-care), playing with family members and other infants/young children (e.g., early education settings), and community experiences (e.g., playground). These deficits are documented by functioning that is 2 standard deviations below the mean in at least two areas of adaptive functioning.

Age: The infant/young child must be at least 6 months old.

Links to DSM–5 and ICD–10

DSM–5: Global Developmental Delay
ICD–10: Other Disorders of Psychological Development, Global Developmental Delay (F88)

10.6 Developmental Language Disorder

Introduction

Developmental Language Disorder is diagnosed when the young child exhibits significant delays in expressive or receptive communication that are not due to sensory impairment (e.g., hearing loss), medical/neurological conditions (e.g., traumatic brain injury or acquired epileptic aphasia), or other neurodevelopmental disorders (e.g., Autism Spectrum Disorder or Global Developmental Delay). Language and communication skills should be selectively impaired in Developmental Language Disorder, even if other delays (e.g., motor or cognitive delays) are present. Often, the etiology of the Developmental Language

Disorder is unknown, although young children with language disorders may have a positive family history for language disorders.

The range of potential language limitations in young children with this disorder is large, ranging from those who exhibit primarily articulation problems to those who exhibit profound delays in understanding spoken language. Although expressive language problems may be identified in the absence of receptive language abnormalities, the reverse is rarely true.

Associated features are varied. Expressive abnormalities may be accompanied by behavioral problems, especially aggressive and angry outbursts. These problems may improve as the young child learns to communicate his or her needs more directly. Alternatively, some young children may adapt to their language delays by becoming more shy and withdrawn. Serious receptive language abnormalities are more challenging to treat than purely expressive delays and have been associated with long-term difficulties in language, learning, and social adaptation. Social abnormalities often accompany serious language impairments, and distinguishing between a primary Developmental Language Disorder and Autism Spectrum Disorder may be challenging.

The later young children are diagnosed with language delays, the worse the prognosis, suggesting that there is an urgency about initiating careful assessment and early intervention. Hearing assessments are always indicated in young children with unexplained language delays. Considering speech, language, and communication developmental milestones must include the young child's cultural and language context. Assessment methods should be valid for the appropriate language and culture. Norms standardized on one group cannot be assumed to be relevant for a different group. Special attention should be paid to young children growing up in bilingual environments because monolingual norms may not apply. A diagnosis of Developmental Language Disorder is made on the basis of history, observation, and performance on standardized tests of language ability.

Diagnostic Algorithm

All of the following criteria must be met.

A. Consistent difficulties or delays in the acquisition and use of language and communication compared with age norms that are characterized by one or more of the following:

   1. Delays in production of gestures, vocalizations, words, or sentences that are significantly below developmental norms. For young children using words, this may include problems using grammatical and morphological rules of language, such as producing novel word combinations, adding tense markers (e.g., "–ing"), and using regular plurals.

   2. Delays in the understanding of gestures, vocalizations, words, phrases, or sentences that are significantly below developmental norms.

   3. Difficulty or delay using language to make needs known, relate experiences, or have a conversation (i.e., impairments in discourse).

B. The language abnormalities described in criterion A are not attributable to the following:

1. Hearing or other sensory impairment, motor dysfunction, or another medical or neurological condition.

2. Another neurodevelopmental disorder.

3. A serious trauma.

C. Deficits in production and understanding of language impair performance of age-expected communication skills. Without supports, the deficits limit the young child's participation and engagement in one or more age-expected activities. These deficits are documented by functioning that is at least 2 standard deviations below the mean on standardized tests.

Age: The young child must be at least 24 months old.

Duration: The symptoms must be present for 3 months.

Links to DSM–5 and ICD–10

DSM–5: Language Disorder
ICD–10: Developmental Disorder of Speech and Language, Unspecified (F80.9)

10.7 Developmental Coordination Disorder

Introduction

Developmental Coordination Disorder (DCD) is diagnosed when the young child exhibits a persistent inability to engage in developmental age-expected coordination of gross and fine motor movements that is not due to a sensory impairment or neurological condition and that is not due to Global Developmental Delay. That is, the motor coordination difficulties are impaired relative to the young child's motor, cognitive, and language status. For this reason, young children with this disorder may or may not also demonstrate developmental delays in major motor milestones. They also are likely to demonstrate reduced abilities to smoothly coordinate other motor demands, such as walking up and down stairs or cutting with scissors. Slowness and awkwardness in motor activities requiring coordination is a notable feature of the disorder.

The diagnosis is made only if the coordination difficulties are functionally impairing for the young child and family, such as interfering with the young child's ability to participate in daily activities requiring motor coordination (e.g., physical games with siblings or peers, getting dressed, using writing implements in preschool or child care).

The onset of this disorder is insidious. A sudden onset following more typical progression in motor coordination skills should lead to a consideration of other conditions. A diagnosis of DCD should not be made in young children less than 24 months old to ensure that young children have adequate opportunity to practice walking and other fine and gross motor skills.

The disorder is more common in males than females. Risk factors include pre-natal alcohol exposure and preterm birth. Some young children with DCD will become sensitive about their perceived deficits and will become socially with-drawn or muted affectively.

As with other neurodevelopmental disorders, early referral for assessment and intervention is indicated. Neurodevelopmental disorders often co-occur, so assessments of DCD should consider the possibility of other neurodevelopmental disorders and vice versa.

Diagnostic Algorithm

All of the following criteria must be met.

A. Coordination of motor skills is markedly below expectations given the young child's mental age and experience with skill acquisition. The young child exhibits at least two of the following symptoms:

1. A pattern of gross and fine motor clumsiness.

2. Clearly demonstrated difficulties with goal-directed motor coordination across multiple settings (e.g., walking across room to get a toy, climbing up on chair).

3. Problems with coordination that affect both speed and accuracy in activities that require sequenced motor skills (e.g., tracking and catching a ball, riding a tricycle, climbing up steps, using crayons).

B. The motor skill deficits are not better explained by Global Developmental Delay, sensory impairments (e.g., visual impairment), or a neurological condition affecting motor coordination (e.g., cerebral palsy or traumatic brain injury).

C. Symptoms of the disorder, or caregiver accommodations in response to the symptoms, significantly affect the young child's and family's functioning in one or more of the following ways:

1. Cause distress to the young child;

2. Interfere with the young child's relationships;

3. Limit the young child's participation in developmentally expected activities or routines;

4. Limit the family's participation in everyday activities or routines; or

5. Limit the young child's ability to learn and develop new skills or interfere with developmental progress.

Age: The diagnosis should not be made in young children less than 24 months old.

Specify:

1. With or without social withdrawal/isolation

2. With or without muted affect

DSM–5: Developmental Coordination Disorder
ICD–10: Specific Developmental Disorder of Motor Function
(Developmental Coordination Disorder) (F82)

10.8 Other Neurodevelopmental Disorder of Infancy/Early Childhood

Diagnostic Algorithm

All of the following criteria must be met.

A. The infant/young child has one or more persistent symptoms of a neurodevelopmental disorder but does not meet full criteria for any disorder in this section.

B. The symptoms are not already encompassed in another disorder for which the infant/young child meets full criteria.

C. Symptoms of the disorder, or caregiver accommodations in response to the symptoms, significantly affect the infant's/young child's and family's functioning in one or more of the following ways:

1. Cause distress to the infant/young child;

2. Interfere with the infant's/young child's relationships;

3. Limit the infant's/young child's participation in developmentally expected activities or routines;

4. Limit the family's participation in everyday activities or routines; or

5. Limit the infant's/young child's ability to learn and develop new skills or interfere with developmental progress.

Specify:

1. The disorder that best explains the infant's/young child's symptoms

2. Why the infant/young child does not meet full criteria

Links to DSM–5 and ICD–10

DSM–5: Unspecified Neurodevelopmental Disorder
ICD–10: Unspecified Disorder of Psychological Development (F89)

20 SENSORY PROCESSING DISORDERS

Sensory processing disorders are diagnosed when the infant/young child demonstrates behaviors that are believed to reflect abnormalities in regulating sensory input. The behaviors cause distress or impair the infant's/young child's functioning in daily activities. Sensory processing disorders affect individuals throughout infancy and early childhood, and there is evidence that these problems are stable in the first years of life.

There is now considerable empirical evidence that some infants/young children experience clinically significant and impairing responses to sensory stimuli that are independent of other psychopathological and neurodevelopmental conditions. These responses may be characterized by over-responsivity (e.g., heightened magnitude of response, faster latency of response, and slower habituation or recovery from response to sensory stimuli), under-responsivity (e.g., reduced magnitude of response, or slower latency to respond to sensory stimuli), or atypical responses to stimuli that may be characterized by extended sensory exploration of stimuli that is typically not noticed (e.g., licking walls or doorknobs). The sensory abnormalities must occur in more than one context (e.g., home, child care, community settings) and may involve one or more sensory domains (e.g., tactile, visual, auditory, vestibular, olfactory, taste, the sense of position of joints or pressure on muscles [proprioceptive sensation], and the sensations from internal organs [interoception]). Failure to process or respond to sensory information in an age-typical manner is associated with impairments for the infant/young child and his or her family.

The symptoms are not better accounted for by another mental disorder (e.g., Attention Deficit Hyperactivity Disorder, Generalized Anxiety Disorder, Autism Spectrum Disorder, or Posttraumatic Stress Disorder) but may co-occur with other mental disorders (with the exception of Autism Spectrum Disorder because atypical sensory responsivity is now a repetitive and restricted behavior criterion).

In contrast to regulatory disorders that were defined in the DC:0–3 and DC:0–3R, the focus on sensory processing disorders is exclusively on over- and under-responsiveness, with an "Other" category for less typical presentations. Difficulties in motor coordination are defined elsewhere and are not included in the criteria.

20.1 Sensory Over-Responsivity Disorder

Introduction

The central feature of Sensory Over-Responsivity Disorder is a persistent pattern of exaggerated, intense, or prolonged responses to sensory stimuli that are more severe, frequent, or enduring than are typically observed in individuals of similar age and developmental level. The sensory over-responsivity occurs in more than one context (e.g., home, child care/preschool, community settings) and can involve one or more sensory domains (e.g., tactile, sound, vision, taste, olfactory, movement through space [vestibular sensation], sense of position of joints or pressure on muscles [proprioceptive sensation], and the sensations from internal organs [interoception]). Although individual differences in sensory sensitivity exist, it is defined as a disorder when there is evidence that the sensory over-responsivity causes significant distress or results in impairment for the infant/young child or his or her family. The sensory over-responsivity symptoms observed are not better accounted for by another mental disorder (e.g., Attention Deficit Hyperactivity Disorder, Generalized Anxiety Disorder, Autism Spectrum Disorder [ASD], or Posttraumatic Stress Disorder [PTSD]) but may co-occur with other mental disorders.

Diagnostic Algorithm

All of the following criteria must be met.

A. The infant/young child displays a persistent and pervasive pattern of sensory over-responsivity that involves intense, negative reactions to one or more types of routine sensory stimuli (including tactile, visual, auditory, vestibular, olfactory, taste, proprioceptive, or interoceptive) in more than one context (e.g., home, child care, playground) and with different caregivers (if the infant/young child has more than one caregiver). The intensity of reactivity or the duration of reactivity is disproportionate to the intensity of the stimulus. Either criterion 1 or 2 below must be present:

1. The infant/young child shows intense emotional or behavioral responses when exposed to stimuli that evoke the sensation. The intensity and duration of the response are disproportionate to the intensity of the stimulus.

2. The infant/young child predictably tries to avoid contact with routine sensory stimuli that are aversive to him or her.

B. The infant/young child does not meet criteria for ASD. Symptoms are not better explained by Attention Deficit Hyperactivity Disorder.

C. Symptoms of the disorder, or caregiver accommodations in response to the symptoms, significantly affect the infant's/young child's and family's functioning in one or more of the following ways:

1. Cause distress to the infant/young child;

2. Interfere with the infant's/young child's relationships;

3. Limit the infant's/young child's participation in developmentally expected activities or routines;

4. Limit the family's participation in everyday activities or routines; or

5. Limit the infant's/young child's ability to learn and develop new skills or interfere with developmental progress.

Age: The infant/young child must be at least 6 months old.

Duration: The pattern of sensory over-responsivity is present for at least 3 months.

Specify:

Tactile: _____ people
                                _____ objects

Auditory: _____a specific kind of noise or decibel level of all noise (e.g., a specific stimulus of everyday life, such as a blender, toilet, or vacuum)

Olfactory: _____

Vestibular: _____ movement in space

Taste: _____ (e.g., spicy foods, bland foods, smooth foods, chewy foods—distinguish from tactile)

Visual: _____ (e.g., bright lights, moving color)

Proprioceptive: _____ cannot judge force appropriately (e.g., pushes too hard without malice, erases through paper)

Interoceptive: _____ sensations from internal organs (e.g., frequent stomach aches)

Diagnostic Features

The central criterion of Sensory Over-Responsivity Disorder is a consistent and persistent pattern of exaggerated, intense, or prolonged responses to sensory stimuli that is more severe, frequent, or enduring than is typically observed in individuals of similar age and developmental level. The sensory over-responsivity occurs in more than one context (e.g., home, child care/preschool, community settings) and can involve one or more sensory domains (e.g., tactile, sound, vision, taste, olfactory, movement through space [vestibular sensation], the sense of position of joints or pressure on muscles [proprioceptive sensation], and the sensations from internal organs [interoception]).

Associated Features Supporting Diagnosis

Evidence from neuroimaging studies indicates that when compared with typically developing infants/young children, infants/young children with Sensory Over-Responsivity Disorder show difficulty processing multimodal stimuli, such as a combination of auditory and visual stimuli. In addition, preliminary data suggest dysfunction of white matter in the posterior part of the brain. To date, this work has not been linked to real-world impairments, but the association of behavioral symptoms and neurobiological abnormalities does provide preliminary validity data about sensory over-responsivity. There is also evidence that sensory over-responsivity shows moderate stability through early childhood and that it is heritable, with identical twins having more similar manifestations of sensory over-responsivity than fraternal twins.

Developmental Features

Infants/young children may show sensory over-responsivity symptoms—for example, crying excessively and having difficulty being soothed after exposure to loud noises or showing a consistent pattern of distress in response to being soothed by tactile, gentle movement (e.g., rocking) or other sensory experiences. As infants/young children get older, they may develop patterns of avoidance or opposition when asked to engage in activities that involve exposure to sensations to which they have adverse responses.

Prevalence

The prevalence of Sensory Over-Responsivity Disorder is unknown, but epidemiological data based on parent report of symptoms suggest prevalence between 5% and 16.5% associated with family impairment.

Course

The course of Sensory Over-Responsivity Disorder is unknown. However, there is moderate stability in Sensory Over-Responsivity Disorder symptoms between 1 and 8 years old, and, on average, all young children show an increase in sensory over-responsivity behaviors between 1 and 3 years old.

Risk and Prognostic Features

Infants who are born preterm or small for gestational age appear to be at elevated risk for Sensory Over-Responsivity Disorder. In addition, environmental conditions—including lack of movement/tactile stimulation in the early years (e.g., due to being raised in an orphanage), exposure to drugs or prenatal stress, cumulative risk, or community violence—appear to increase risk for Sensory Over-Responsivity Disorder. Furthermore, infants/young children with Global Developmental Delays or intellectual disabilities are at increased risk for Sensory Over-Responsivity Disorder. Finally, Sensory Over-Responsivity Disorder symptoms appear to be heritable.

Culture-Related Diagnostic Issues

As there is cultural variation in recognition of somatic symptoms across cultures, an infant's/young child's sensory symptoms must be evaluated in the context of the infant's/young child's family and community cultural beliefs and practices.

Gender-Related Diagnostic Issues

There are no known gender differences in rates of Sensory Over-Responsivity Disorder.

Differential Diagnosis

Given that atypical sensory responsivity is now a criterion for ASD, it is not possible to diagnose both ASD and Sensory Over-Responsivity Disorder. It is necessary to determine if sensory over-responsivity is not better explained by PTSD or Other Trauma, Stress, and Deprivation Disorder. In addition, it can be challenging to distinguish some anxiety responses from sensory responses (e.g., fear of vacuum cleaner). If the infant/young child is only bothered by one loud object, it is unlikely that the source of the distress reflects a sensory abnormality. It is critical to observe a pattern of sensory over-responsivity that occurs across settings and stimuli that share a sensory component.

Comorbidity

The majority of infants/young children with Sensory Over-Responsivity Disorder do not have co-occurring psychiatric diagnoses. Infants with Sensory Over-Responsivity Disorder can manifest severe feeding problems, sleep problems, and difficulties with self-soothing. In preschool, young children with Sensory Over-Responsivity Disorder are at elevated risk for emotional and behavior problems, and school-age children are more likely to have academic difficulties. There appears to be a very high risk of anxiety disorders among infants/young children with Sensory Over-Responsivity Disorder, and parents of young children with Obsessive Compulsive Disorder report extremely high rates of sensory over-responsivity.

Links to DSM–5 and ICD–10

DSM–5: Other Specified Neurodevelopmental Disorder
ICD–10: Other Disorders of Psychological Development (F88)

20.2 Sensory Under-Responsivity Disorder

Introduction

The central feature of Sensory Under-Responsivity Disorder is a persistent pattern of muted, minimal, neutral, or extremely brief responses to sensory stimuli that is not consistent with developmental expectations. The sensory under-responsivity occurs in more than one context (e.g., home, child care/preschool, community settings) and can involve one or more sensory domains (e.g., tactile, sound, vision, taste, olfactory, movement through space [vestibular sensation], the sense of position of joints or pressure on muscles [proprioceptive sensation], and the sensations from internal organs [interoception]). Because individual differences in sensory responsiveness exist, sensory under-responsivity behaviors are defined as a disorder when there is clear evidence that the sensory under-responsivity causes significant distress or results in impairment for the infant/young child or his or her family. The sensory under-responsivity symptoms observed are not better accounted for by another mental disorder (e.g., Attention Deficit Hyperactivity Disorder [ADHD] inattentive type, depression, Autism Spectrum Disorder [ASD]) but may co-occur with other mental disorders other than ASD.

Diagnostic Algorithm

All of the following criteria must be met.

A. The infant/young child displays a persistent and pervasive pattern of sensory under-responsivity that involves muted or neutral reactions to one or more types of intense sensory stimuli (including tactile, visual, auditory, vestibular, olfactory, or taste) in more than one context (e.g., home, child care/school, playground) and with different caregivers (if the infant/young child has more than one caregiver). The minimal intensity of reactivity or the latency to initiate a response is disproportionate to the intensity of the stimulus. Either criterion 1 or 2 below must be present:

1. The infant/young child shows muted emotional or behavioral responses when exposed to intense stimuli that are expected to evoke a strong or at least a moderate sensory response. The minimal intensity of reactivity, long latency to respond, and brief duration of the response are disproportionate to the intensity of the stimulus.

2. The infant/young child is predictably unresponsive to routine sensory stimuli that would be expected to evoke a strong positive or aversive response (even when the lack of response may be associated with injury).

B. Symptoms of the disorder, or caregiver accommodations in response to the symptoms, significantly affect the infant's/young child's and family's functioning in one or more of the following ways:

1. Cause distress to the infant/young child;

2. Interfere with the infant's/young child's relationships;

3. Limit the infant's/young child's participation in developmentally expected activities or routines;

4. Limit the family's participation in everyday activities or routines; or

5. Limit the infant's/young child's ability to learn and develop new skills or interfere with developmental progress.

Age: The infant/young child must be at least 6 months old.

Duration: The pattern of sensory under-responsivity is present for at least 3 months.

Specify:

Tactile:	_____	people
	_____	objects
Auditory:	_____	a specific kind of noise or decibel level of all noise
Olfactory:	_____	
Vestibular:	_____	movement in space
Taste:	_____	(distinguish from tactile)
Visual:	_____	(e.g., bright lights, moving colors)
Proprioceptive:	_____	(sense of body based on input from muscles)
Interoceptive:	_____	(sensations from internal organs)

Diagnostic Features

The central criterion of Sensory Under-Responsivity Disorder is a consistent and persistent pattern of muted, minimal, or extremely brief responses to sensory stimuli that is much less intense, frequent, or enduring than is typically observed in individuals of similar age and developmental level. The sensory under-responsivity occurs in more than one context (e.g., home, child care/preschool, community settings) and can involve one or more sensory domains (e.g., tactile, sound, vision, taste, olfactory, movement through space [vestibular sensation], the sense of position of joints or pressure on muscles [proprioceptive sensation], and the sensations from internal organs [interoception]). For example, the infant/young child may be unaware of pain even when bloodied by a fall or may not notice a television being turned on at a very loud volume.

Associated Features Supporting Diagnosis

There are no known associated features for Sensory Under-Responsivity Disorder.

Developmental Features

There are no known developmental differences during early childhood in young children with Sensory Under-Responsivity Disorder, but the young child's ability to understand and to communicate about reduced responsiveness increases through the preschool years.

Prevalence

The prevalence of Sensory Under-Responsivity Disorder is unknown, but it is believed to be rare.

Course

The course of Sensory Under-Responsivity Disorder is unknown.

Risk and Prognostic Features

There is not clear evidence regarding risk and prognostic features for Sensory Under-Responsivity Disorder.

Culture-Related Diagnostic Issues

As there are cultural variations in recognition of somatic symptoms across cultures, an infant's/young child's sensory symptoms must be evaluated in the context of his or her family's and community's cultural beliefs and practices.

Gender-Related Diagnostic Issues

There are no known gender differences in rates of Sensory Under-Responsivity Disorder.

Differential Diagnosis

Given that atypical sensory responsivity is a criterion for ASD, the presence of ASD precludes a diagnosis of Sensory Under-Responsivity Disorder. In addition, it can be challenging to distinguish the inattentive type of ADHD from Sensory Under-Responsivity (e.g., failing to respond when a television is turned up very loud). If other symptoms of ADHD can explain the symptoms of under-responsivity, a diagnosis of ADHD should be assigned. Sensory Under-Responsivity Disorder requires clear evidence of limited responsivity to sensory inputs specifically. These infants/young children should also be evaluated for medical conditions in which infants/young children are insensitive to pain.

Comorbidity

There are no data on comorbidities for infants/young children with Sensory Under-Responsivity Disorder.

Links to DSM–5 and ICD–10

DSM–5: Other Specified Neurodevelopmental Disorder
ICD–10: Other Disorders of Psychological Development (F88)

20.3 Other Sensory Processing Disorder

Diagnostic Algorithm

All of the following criteria must be met.

A. The infant/young child displays a persistent and pervasive pattern of atypical sensory responding that does not meet criteria for Sensory Over-Responsivity Disorder or Sensory Under-Responsivity Disorder.

B. The infant's/young child's symptoms are specifically related to sensory stimulation, and the infant/young child does not meet criteria for Autism Spectrum Disorder; furthermore, the symptoms are not better explained by Attention Deficit Hyperactivity Disorder.

C. Symptoms of the disorder, or caregiver accommodations in response to the symptoms, significantly affect the infant's/young child's and family's functioning in one or more of the following ways:

1. Cause distress to the infant/young child;

2. Interfere with the infant's/young child's relationships;

3. Limit the infant's/young child's participation in developmentally expected activities or routines;

4. Limit the family's participation in everyday activities or routines; or

5. Limit the infant's/young child's ability to learn and develop new skills or interfere with developmental progress.

Age: The infant/young child must be at least 6 months old.

Duration: The pattern of sensory over-responsivity or under-responsivity is present for at least 3 months.

Specify:

Tactile: _____ people

_____ objects

Auditory: _____a specific kind of noise or decibel level of all noise

Olfactory: _____

Vestibular: _____ movement in space

Taste: _____ (distinguish from tactile)

Visual: _____ (e.g., bright lights, moving colors)

Proprioceptive: _____ (sense of body based on input from muscles)

Interoceptive: _____ (sensations from internal organs)

Links to DSM–5 and ICD–10

DSM–5: Other Specified Neurodevelopmental Disorder
ICD–10: Other Disorders of Psychological Development (F88)

30 ANXIETY DISORDERS

Until recently, distressing anxiety in infants/young children was regarded either as a normative phase of development or a temperament style imparting risk for anxiety disorders, depression, and other mental health disorders later in life. It is now clear that early childhood anxiety and associated symptoms can reach clinically significant levels, cause significant impairment in infants/young children and their families, and increase risk for anxiety and depression later in childhood and adulthood. Moreover, anxiety disorders in infants/young children, as in older children and adults, present as specific disorders that include Separation Anxiety Disorder, Social Phobia, Generalized Anxiety Disorder, and Specific Phobias.

Identifying clinically significant anxiety and specific anxiety disorders in infants/young children is challenging. Older children and adults are better able than infants/young children to verbally describe their internal experiences and emotions, including fear, anxiety, and worry. Thus, assessment of anxiety in early childhood depends on descriptions of the infant's/young child's emotional state that (1) are based on the infant's/young child's behaviors and manifest distress and (2) are primarily based on adult report (e.g., parent, teacher/child care provider) or observational assessments (e.g., structured observations at home/school or child care). Young children who are 3 years old and older may verbalize their anxiety and fears and represent these internal experiences within their play.

The symptom presentations for specific anxiety disorders in early childhood are remarkably similar to symptoms at older ages, although symptom manifestation clearly differs by age. Anxiety disorders must be distinguished from developmentally typical anxiety/fears. Several general criteria must be met for an infant's/young child's anxiety or fears to be considered as a possible symptom of an anxiety disorder: The anxiety symptoms must (1) cause the infant/young child distress, or lead to avoidance of activities or settings associated with the anxiety or fear; (2) occur during two or more everyday activities, or within two or more relationships; (3) be uncontrollable, at least some of the time; (4) persist for at least 2 weeks (note that for some disorders, the duration is longer than 2 weeks); (5) impair the infant's/young child's or the family's functioning; and (6) impair the infant's/young child's expected development.

Because the majority of research on anxiety disorders groups Separation Anxiety Disorder, Social Anxiety Disorder, and Generalized Anxiety Disorder together, the text for these three disorders is presented together with distinctions between disorders noted when known. Following that are criteria and text for Selective Mutism, Inhibition to Novelty Disorder, and Other Anxiety Disorder of Infancy/Early Childhood.

30.1 Separation Anxiety Disorder

Diagnostic Algorithm

All of the following criteria must be met.

A. The infant/young child displays developmentally inappropriate and excessive signs of anxiety concerning separation from home or from those to whom the infant/young child is attached. At least some of the time, the infant/young child cannot regulate the anxiety even with external reassurance. The anxiety is evidenced by at least three of the following seven symptoms:

1. Recurrent, excessive distress when separation from home or major attachment figures occurs or is anticipated.

2. Persistent, excessive worry that some event (e.g., getting lost or being kidnapped) will lead to separation from a major attachment figure. Preverbal or barely verbal infants/young children have limited abilities to express worries.

3. Persistent reluctance or refusal to go to child care, school, or other settings outside the home because of fear of separation. This may appear as (a) fear or anxiety related to leaving home for child care or school; (b) anticipatory fear or anxiety related to child care or school; (c) resisting or refusing to go to child care or school because of fear or anxiety; or (d) crying, clinging, hiding, tantrums, or other efforts to avoid separation. Infants/young children may express their anxiety/fear with inconsolable crying or clinging.

4. Persistent or excessive fear or reluctance to be alone or without major attachment figures at home or without significant adult caregivers in other settings.

5. Persistent reluctance or refusal to go to sleep without the presence of a major attachment figure for at least 1 month.

6. Repeated nightmares involving the theme of separation. Preverbal or barely verbal infants/young children may have frightening dreams without recognizable content.

7. Physical or physiological symptoms when separation from major attachment figures occurs or is anticipated.

B. Symptoms of the disorder, or caregiver accommodations in response to the symptoms, significantly affect the infant's/young child's and family's functioning in one or more of the following ways:

1. Cause distress to the infant/young child;

2. Interfere with the infant's/young child's relationships;

3. Limit the infant's/young child's participation in developmentally expected activities or routines;

4. Limit the family's participation in everyday activities or routines; or

5. Limit the infant's/young child's ability to learn and develop new skills or interfere with developmental progress.

Duration: The fear, anxiety, or avoidance is persistent, typically lasting for at least 1 month.

Links to DSM–5 and ICD–10

DSM–5: Separation Anxiety Disorder
ICD–10: Separation Anxiety Disorder of Childhood (F93.0)

30.2 Social Anxiety Disorder (Social Phobia)

Diagnostic Algorithm

All of the following criteria must be met. Criteria can be met if the young child has demonstrated these behaviors in the past and exposure is currently avoided or intentionally limited by caregivers.

A. The young child exhibits marked and persistent fear of one or more social or performance situations that involve exposure to unfamiliar people or possible scrutiny by others commonly shown with peers and adults. The fear or anxiety is out of proportion to the threat posed by the social situation.

B. Exposure to the feared social situation almost invariably provokes anxiety in the young child, who may express anxiety by panicking, crying, tantruming, freezing, clinging, shrinking, or failing to speak in social situations with unfamiliar people.

C. The young child avoids the feared social or performance situation(s) or endures it with intense anxiety or distress.

D. The fear is not better accounted for by other disorders, including Autism Spectrum Disorder, Separation Anxiety Disorder, or other anxiety disorders.

E. Symptoms of the disorder, or caregiver accommodations in response to the symptoms, significantly affect the young child's and family's functioning in one or more of the following ways:

1. Cause distress to the young child;

2. Interfere with the young child's relationships;

3. Limit the young child's participation in developmentally expected activities or routines;

4. Limit the family's participation in everyday activities or routines; or

5. Limit the young child's ability to learn and develop new skills or interfere with developmental progress.

Age: The young child is at least 24 months old.

Duration: The symptoms must be present for 2 months or more.

Links to DSM–5 and ICD–10

DSM–5: Social Anxiety Disorder (Social Phobia)
ICD–10: Social Anxiety Disorder of Childhood (F93.2)

30.3 Generalized Anxiety Disorder

Diagnostic Algorithm

All of the following criteria must be met.

A. The young child experiences marked and persistent anxiety or worry more days than not. Worries may include anxiety about future events, the appropriateness of past behavior, and concern about competence in one or more areas.

B. The young child is unable to regulate the anxiety or worry (e.g., the young child may repeatedly ask a parent for reassurance).

C. The anxiety and worry occur during two or more activities or settings or within two or more relationships.

D. The anxiety and worry are associated with one or more of the following six symptoms:

1. Agitation

2. Fatigability

3. Intermittent inattention

4. Irritability (e.g., easily frustrated)

5. Muscle tension and difficulty relaxing

6. Sleep disturbance (e.g., difficulty falling or staying asleep; restless, unsatisfying sleep; or being awakened by scary dreams)

E. The anxiety or worry is generalized and not limited to the worries that are found in Obsessive Compulsive Disorder (e.g., fears of contamination), Posttraumatic Stress Disorder (e.g., anxiety about people or places following a trauma), Separation Anxiety Disorder (e.g., anxiety about separation from a caregiver), or Social Anxiety Disorder (e.g., worry about social interactions).

F. The disturbance is not due to the direct physiologic effect of a substance (e.g., asthma medication or steroids).

G. Symptoms of the disorder, or caregiver accommodations in response to the symptoms, significantly affect the young child's and family's functioning in one or more of the following ways:

1. Cause distress to the young child;

2. Interfere with the young child's relationships;

3. Limit the young child's participation in developmentally expected activities or routines;

4. Limit the family's participation in everyday activities or routines; or

5. Limit the young child's ability to learn and develop new skills or interfere with developmental progress.

Age: The diagnosis should be made with caution in young children less than 36 months old.

Duration: The symptoms must be present for at least 2 months.

Diagnostic Features

The most significant barrier to identification and treatment of young children with impairing anxiety is the widespread belief among many adult caregivers that young children can control their anxiety and associated behaviors and will outgrow their symptoms. In addition, identifying these disorders requires adult caregivers to make inferences about the internal feeling states of young children.

Separation Anxiety Disorder, Generalized Anxiety Disorder, and Social Phobia each present with constellations of symptoms that are relatively similar to those found in older children and adults. The anxious distress that is common to all three anxiety disorders may manifest in young children as inconsolable crying, clinging, hiding, reactive tantrums, or other behaviors that reflect the young child's efforts to avoid a perceived threat.

The perceived threat differs among the anxiety disorders. For Separation Anxiety Disorder, the perceived threat is actual or anticipated separation from the young child's primary caregiver. Unfamiliar people and situations are perceived as threatening in Social Phobia. Most of the symptoms of these two disorders describe behaviors that can be observed. The hallmark of Generalized Anxiety Disorder is worry—an anxiety state that is not provoked by an immediate perceived threat but rather is linked to worries about the past and anticipatory anxiety about the future. Worry, an internal anxiety state, can be difficult to identify in young children, particularly young children who are developing their capacities to express their emotions and thoughts verbally.

To be considered clinically significant, each symptom must have all of these characteristics: The anxiety must be intense (excessive distress), uncontrollable (does not decrease with reassurance or repetition), recurrent, developmentally inappropriate, and persistent (occurs for more than 1 month). If the symptom threshold for a specific anxiety disorder is met, then the young child's and family's functioning must also be affected.

Attempting to avoid anxiety-provoking situations/triggers is a common response for individuals of any age with impairing anxiety. This strategy for alleviating anxiety often leads to maladaptive symptoms that adversely affect development and functioning. For young children with anxiety, parents may facilitate this avoidance. For example, it is not uncommon for parents of young children with Separation Anxiety Disorder to develop routines that allow the young child to avoid separation and thus avoid experiencing separation symptoms. The young child might not attend preschool or child care, may sleep in the parents' bed despite the parents' wish that the young child sleep independently, and may never be left in the care of anyone other than the parents. In these cases, the clinician has to assess how the young child would respond if he or she was faced with separation.

Associated Features Supporting Diagnosis

Heightened physiological arousal (e.g., increased heart rate, blinking, sweating, dizziness, and muscle tension) is a common associated feature of anxiety disorders. In young children, stomach aches and headaches are also common. Understanding the link between emotions and the body's responses to and expressions of emotions is critical both for assessment of the young child's symptoms as well as choice of interventions. Temper tantrums and other types of dysregulated behavior are also commonly associated with early childhood anxiety disorders. It is critical that these behaviors be evaluated within the broad context of the young child's emotion regulation capacities and functioning and be understood as one of the common ways that young children respond to and express their emotional distress.

Developmental Features

A critical challenge for clinicians and researchers is defining the difference between developmentally appropriate anxiety and developmentally inappropriate and excessive anxiety. For example, stranger anxiety and separation anxiety are developmentally typical in infancy. They reflect evolutionary selection of an infant's/young child's adaptive response to unfamiliar adults and being alone— threats that potentially reflect danger to the infant/young child. Normative fears and anxiety peak at 3 years old. For the majority of young children, these anxieties and fear responses are transient and do not derail the young child's cognitive, social, or emotional development. Understanding that young children's emotional and social capacities are developing concurrently with the young child's physical, cognitive, and verbal capacities is the foundation necessary to identify atypical and impairing anxiety disorders.

For example, distress in response to separation from the primary caregiver (separation anxiety) is a typical developmental stage that usually emerges at about 8 months old and subsides by 24 months old. The peak for many infants/young children is 10–18 months old. Separation anxiety at this stage is a reflection of both the infant's/young child's attachment to his or her primary caregiver(s) and emerging cognitive understanding that people and objects exist even if they are not present. Young children's understanding of time emerges later, so they do not yet understand when or even if a parent will ever come back. For this reason, studies of Separation Anxiety Disorder in young children have begun at 2 years old or older. With young children less than 2 years old, the intensity and pervasiveness of the separation anxiety and associated impairment may raise concern that should be addressed even if the infant/young child does not meet full criteria for a disorder.

The clinician must also account for temperamental variation in the assessment of anxiety disorders in infants/young children. Behaviorally inhibited infants/ young children demonstrate characteristics that have been shown to be associated with increased risk for anxiety disorders, depression, and other disorders later in childhood. However, these temperamental characteristics are not always associated with other anxiety symptoms or predictive of impairment, although young children with behaviorally inhibited temperaments/shyness also can meet criteria for an anxiety disorder. Research suggests that Social Anxiety Disorder can reliably be identified in young children more than 2 years old. There is overlap between the symptoms of Social Anxiety Disorder and behavioral inhibition; a Social Anxiety Disorder diagnosis requires that each of the symptoms meets the criteria established to distinguish between typical and atypical presentations (e.g., severity, persistence) and must co-occur with impairment.

Because of the difficulty of identifying the internal state of worry in young children with limited verbal capacities, Generalized Anxiety Disorder has not been commonly studied or identified in young children less than 3 years old. Research in older children and preschoolers suggests that Generalized Anxiety Disorder may be more closely related to depression, which has been shown to present as early as 2 years old.

Prevalence

Early childhood anxiety symptoms and disorders represent a major mental health problem, with prevalence for any anxiety disorder in epidemiological studies ranging from 9% to 20%. Rates for each type of anxiety disorder range from ~2% to 10% without significant difference in rates between Social Phobia, Separation Anxiety Disorder, and Generalized Anxiety Disorder. These rates are consistent with the rates of anxiety disorders in later childhood and adulthood.

Course

The persistence and course of early childhood anxiety disorders are similar to that at older ages. Early anxiety disorders increase a young child's risk for anxiety disorders, as well as depression and Disruptive Behavior Disorder, at school age and adolescence. Early childhood anxiety disorders also increase the chance that the young child's functioning will be impaired, particularly in the social realm, as the young child progresses through childhood.

Risk and Prognostic Features

Most studies of risk factors for early childhood anxiety disorders aggregate anxiety disorders together rather than examine specific anxiety disorders. Risk factors associated with impairing anxiety in early childhood include prenatal factors (e.g., maternal smoking during pregnancy), family history (e.g., family history of anxiety and depression), parent factors (e.g., maternal depression), young child characteristics (e.g., behavioral inhibition, shyness, heightened startle reaction), parenting styles (e.g., parental overprotection, coercive parenting), family structure (e.g., increased number of siblings, single parenting), environmental factors (e.g., exposure to violence, particularly domestic violence), adverse life experiences (e.g., medical illnesses requiring hospitalizations and procedures), and demographic factors (e.g., economic adversity).

Culture-Related Diagnostic Issues

No cultural differences in the specific clinical picture of Separation Anxiety Disorder, Social Anxiety Disorder, or Generalized Anxiety Disorder have been demonstrated in young children, although culturally different expectations and practices can affect the assessment of whether symptoms are typical or atypical. In cultures that proscribe eye contact as a way of showing respect, young children may appear to be shy even if they are not. The common practice of young children and parents sharing a bed should not be automatically identified as a symptom of separation anxiety, as co-sleeping is common in many cultures and subcultures.

Gender-Related Diagnostic Issues

Some studies have suggested that girls have higher rates of anxiety disorders, particularly Separation Anxiety Disorder; however, other studies have found no difference by gender.

Differential Diagnosis

Because the symptoms of anxiety disorders in young children overlap with symptoms of other disorders (e.g., irritability in Generalized Anxiety Disorder and depression) and associated features (e.g., temper tantrums), careful assessment and consideration of differential diagnoses are critical. Other mental health disorders, including depression and Posttraumatic Stress Disorder, should be considered (and may be comorbid). Delirium, commonly found in neonatal and pediatric intensive care units, must be ruled out. Other medical conditions to be considered include migraines, seizure disorders, central nervous system disorders, respiratory disorders, and sleep disorders. Medication-induced anxiety (e.g., asthma medication, corticosteroids, antivirals) should also be ruled out. Drug intoxication (e.g., unintentional ingestion of analgesics containing caffeine) should also be considered.

Comorbidity

The concurrent comorbidity pattern for anxiety disorders in young children is somewhat different than the pattern for older children. First, more than two thirds of young children with an anxiety disorder meet criteria for one anxiety disorder, whereas "pure" anxiety disorders seem to be less common in older children. Other studies have shown that when anxiety disorders are considered as a single group, depression and Disruptive Behavior Disorder—in addition to other anxiety disorders—are more likely to co-occur. One population study of comorbidity associated with specific anxiety disorders found different patterns by disorder: (a) Generalized Anxiety Disorder was significantly associated with Separation Anxiety Disorder, Social Anxiety Disorder, depression, and Disruptive Behavior Disorder; (b) Separation Anxiety Disorder was significantly associated with Generalized Anxiety Disorder alone; and (c) Social Anxiety Disorder was associated with Generalized Anxiety Disorder and Attention Deficit Hyperactivity Disorder.

Young children with anxiety disorders are also more likely to have hypersensitivity to sensory stimuli (e.g., noise, smells, tastes) and to be "picky eaters." Anxiety disorders may also be associated with medical conditions including atopic disorders, such as eczema, asthma, and functional abdominal pain. Rates of anxiety disorders are high (>40%) in young children with Autism Spectrum Disorder and genetic disorders, including DiGeorge syndrome.

Links to DSM–5 and ICD–10

DSM–5: Generalized Anxiety Disorder
ICD–10: Generalized Anxiety Disorder (F41.1)

30.4 Selective Mutism

Introduction

Young children with Selective Mutism fail to speak in some situations and to speak normally in other situations. The core symptom is a failure to speak rather than an inability to speak. Selective Mutism presents in early childhood, is persistent, and is highly impairing. Selective Mutism is also highly correlated with both behaviorally inhibited temperaments and symptoms of Social Anxiety Disorder. Although not as common as the other major anxiety disorders, Selective Mutism is highly distressing and is often a severe anxiety disorder. Untreated, Selective Mutism persists and causes significant disruption in the young child's social and emotional development.

Diagnostic Algorithm

All of the following criteria must be met.

A. Consistent failure to speak in specific social situations in which there is an expectation for speaking (e.g., at preschool) despite being able to speak in other situations.

B. Reluctance to speak is not explained by unfamiliarity with the spoken language or expressive language disorder.

C. Symptoms of the disorder, or caregiver accommodations in response to the symptoms, significantly affect the young child's and family's functioning in one or more of the following ways:

1. Cause distress to the young child;

2. Interfere with the young child's relationships;

3. Limit the young child's participation in developmentally expected activities or routines;

4. Limit the family's participation in everyday activities or routines; or

5. Limit the young child's ability to learn and develop new skills or interfere with developmental progress.

Duration: The symptoms must be present for at least 1 month.

Diagnostic Features

Young children with Selective Mutism are capable of speaking and understanding verbal language. A young child with Selective Mutism might speak rarely or might be silent in one setting (e.g., school) and talkative in other settings (e.g., home). The mutism must be present for at least 1 month and cause impairment in the young child and family.

Associated Features Supporting Diagnosis

Previously, Selective Mutism was understood as an elective oppositional behavior rather than emerging from severe anxiety. Associated features reflect that Selective Mutism is a highly impairing anxiety disorder. Social avoidance, social distress, and fear of speaking to unfamiliar people are commonly associated with Selective Mutism. Young children with Selective Mutism might also show other characteristics of impairing anxiety, including a flat facial expression with little smiling, lack of eye contact, extreme shyness, tantrums, difficulty with change, sleep difficulties, and depressed or irritable mood. Physical symptoms such as stomach aches, headaches, and nausea commonly present. Sensory sensitivity is also common.

Developmental Features

Behaviorally inhibited temperament characteristics are significantly associated with Selective Mutism, with the intensity of behavioral inhibition greater for young children with Selective Mutism compared with young children with other emotional disorders. The greater the intensity of the young child's behavioral inhibition, the fewer words that are spoken.

Prevalence

Selective Mutism is an uncommon disorder, with reported prevalence rates ranging from 0.03% to 0.08%.

Course

The mean age of onset is usually between 3 and 4 years old, although diagnosis is commonly made at school age. The mean duration of the disorder is 8 years. Talking behaviors over time remain lower than average for young children with a history of Selective Mutism. Even with the resolution of Selective Mutism, young children often have persistent shyness and social anxiety in adolescence and adulthood. Even with remission, young children with a history of Selective Mutism continue to have communication problems, continue to have increased rates of psychiatric disorders, and are impaired in their academic and social functioning.

Risk and Prognostic Features

Young children with Selective Mutism are more likely to have relatives with Social Anxiety Disorder and relatives with Selective Mutism. Behavioral inhibition is also a risk factor. Immigration has been linked to Selective Mutism. Predictors of ongoing Selective Mutism symptoms and comorbid psychiatric disorders include immigrant status, increased severity of behavioral inhibition and of Selective Mutism, longer duration of mutism, and older age at diagnosis.

Culture-Related Diagnostic Issues

No cultural, racial, or ethnic differences have been identified for Selective Mutism. One study found that young children with Selective Mutism are more likely to live in bilingual or multilingual homes.

Gender-Related Diagnostic Issues

Studies have found that Selective Mutism is more common in girls than boys.

Differential Diagnosis

It is critical to determine that the young child's mutism cannot be better explained by other causes or disorders. Lack of understanding of language or lack of language skills should be ruled out. A primary communication disorder (e.g., social [pragmatic] communication disorder) could be the cause of the young child's mutism. Mutism that occurs in the context of Autism Spectrum Disorder would also rule out Selective Mutism as the cause of the young child's silence. Young children with Selective Mutism can be misdiagnosed with Autism Spectrum Disorder because in both disorders young children present with mutism and social withdrawal. However, young children with Selective Mutism do not present with the repetitive behaviors and social deficits that characterize Autism Spectrum Disorder. Similarly, mutism that presents suddenly after a major traumatic event should be identified as traumatic mutism, not Selective Mutism.

Comorbidity

The most common comorbid disorder for young children with Selective Mutism is Social Anxiety Disorder, with 90%–100% of young children with Selective Mutism meeting criteria for Social Anxiety Disorder. Selective Mutism is also associated with other anxiety disorders as well as nonanxiety disorders, including depression and Obsessive Compulsive Disorder. Although clinically significant behavior problems do present with Selective Mutism, comorbidity with Disruptive Behavior Disorder is relatively uncommon. About 40% of young children with Selective Mutism have speech and language problems (e.g., stuttering, lisps, articulation difficulties, cleft lip); furthermore, in one study, about 70% of young children also met criteria for developmental delays.

Links to DSM–5 and ICD–10

DSM–5: Selective Mutism
ICD–10: Selective Mutism (F94.0)

30.5 Inhibition to Novelty Disorder

Introduction

In contrast to slow-to-warm-up or behaviorally inhibited temperaments that have been described as normal variants of individual dispositions, Inhibition to Novelty Disorder defines extremes of behavioral inhibition that impair the infant's/young child's functioning. Infants/young children with this disorder are commonly referred to primary care providers and to infant/young child mental health clinicians. This disorder appears to increase risk for later emerging anxiety disorders, such as Generalized Anxiety Disorder and Social Anxiety Disorder. Infants/young children with Inhibition to Novelty Disorder show an overall and pervasive difficulty to approach new situations, toys, activities, and persons, which causes distress and interferes with relationships or participation in developmentally expected activities and routines.

Diagnostic Algorithm

All of the following criteria must be met.

A. The infant/young child exhibits fearful symptoms in the presence of novel/unfamiliar objects (e.g., toys), people, and situations. The infant/young child almost always does the following:

1. Freezes or withdraws (e.g., stops vocalizing, avoids eye contact) and attempts to distance him- or herself from the novel object, person, or experience by hiding or seeking the caregiver.

2. Displays marked, persistent, and pervasive negative affect.

B. The inhibited behavior is not better explained as a trauma or stress-related symptom as in Posttraumatic Stress Disorder or Adjustment Disorder and is not simply a phobic reaction to specific stimuli.

C. Symptoms of the disorder, or caregiver accommodations in response to the symptoms, significantly affect the infant's/young child's and family's functioning in one or more of the following ways:

1. Cause distress to the infant/young child;

2. Interfere with the infant's/young child's relationships;

3. Limit the infant's/young child's participation in developmentally expected activities or routines;

4. Limit the family's participation in everyday activities or routines; or

5. Limit the infant's/young child's ability to learn and develop new skills or interfere with developmental progress.

Age: The infant/young child must be less than 24 months old.

Duration: The symptoms of the disorder must be present for at least 1 month.

Diagnostic Features

The essential feature of Inhibition to Novelty Disorder is that infants/young children exhibit fearful symptoms when confronted with new people or situations that are not better explained by a traumatic or frightening event. This fear and inhibition are extreme and associated with impairments in the infant's/young child's and family's functioning. The main functional consequence of the disorder is the restriction of the infant's/young child's exploratory behavior and learning through new experiences and resistance to efforts to encourage exploration.

Associated Features Supporting Diagnosis

Infants/young children with Inhibition to Novelty Disorder appear to be extremely shy and may exhibit negative emotionality.

Developmental Features

Behavioral inhibition has been demonstrated in the second year of life. Some precursors of behavioral inhibition in the first few months of life have been described, but it is unlikely that criteria for this disorder can be met until the latter half of the second year of life. Beyond 24 months old, the disorder is not diagnosed because young children who remain symptomatic after this age seem to display symptoms of other anxiety disorders (e.g., Generalized Anxiety Disorder, Social Anxiety Disorder).

Prevalence

Behavioral inhibition is demonstrable in about 15% of infants/young children. Although no formal data on prevalence of Inhibition to Novelty Disorder have been reported, it represents a small percentage of those with behavioral inhibition.

Course

Behavioral inhibition in infants/young children shows continuity with social wariness at older ages. There are few data regarding the course of Inhibition to Novelty Disorder. It is believed that Inhibition to Novelty Disorder is a precursor of other anxiety disorders that become more clearly manifest at 2–3 years old.

Risk and Prognostic Features

Infants/young children of parents with anxiety disorders are at increased risk for behavioral inhibition and Inhibition to Novelty Disorder. Early manifestations of fearfulness are predictive of other anxiety symptoms emerging in later childhood. Parental shielding of infants/young children from novel experiences increases risk for anxiety symptoms in later childhood. Some inhibited infants/young children continue to display the tendency to withdraw from new stimuli, and they may become less assertive and more prone to rejection than their peers, thus catalyzing the growth of negative self-perceptions. Compared with their peers, infants/young children with behavioral inhibition experience more social rejection, interpret ambiguous social encounters as particularly rejecting, more vigorously tend to avoid social stressors, and more often respond to social rejection with attributions of internal failures and avoidant coping.

Culture-Related Diagnostic Issues

No specific data are available regarding cultural differences, although cultural norms about behavior in familiar and unfamiliar environments and with familiar and unfamiliar people are important to consider.

Gender-Related Diagnostic Issues

No specific data are available regarding gender differences.

Differential Diagnosis

The first consideration is whether the infant's/young child's behavioral inhibition is extreme enough to justify a diagnosis of Inhibition to Novelty Disorder. This is determined by documenting that the anxiety and inhibition cause impairment in the infant's/young child's functioning. Infants/young children may exhibit phobic responses to specific objects, people, or situations, but Inhibition to Novelty Disorder is distinguished by the pervasiveness of situations in which the fearfulness is manifest. Posttraumatic Stress Disorder and Adjustment Disorder may include fearful reactions and freezing behavior, but they follow exposure to a trauma or significant stressor.

Comorbidity

Anxiety disorders tend to co-occur, but in this age range, most other anxiety disorders are challenging to diagnose. No other comorbidities are known.

Links to DSM–5 and ICD–10

DSM–5: Other Specified Anxiety Disorder
ICD–10: Other Specified Anxiety Disorder (F41.8)

30.6 Other Anxiety Disorder of Infancy/Early Childhood

Diagnostic Algorithm

All of the following criteria must be met.

A. The infant/young child has one or more persistent symptoms of an anxiety disorder but does not meet full criteria for any disorder in this section.

B. The symptoms are not already encompassed in another disorder for which the infant/young child meets full criteria.

C. Symptoms of the disorder, or caregiver accommodations in response to the symptoms, significantly affect the infant's/young child's and family's functioning in one or more of the following ways:

    1. Cause distress to the infant/young child;

    2. Interfere with the infant's/young child's relationships;

3. Limit the infant's/young child's participation in developmentally expected activities or routines;

4. Limit the family's participation in everyday activities or routines; or

5. Limit the infant's/young child's ability to learn and develop new skills or interfere with developmental progress.

Specify:

1. The disorder that best explains the infant's/young child's symptoms

2. Why the infant/young child does not meet full criteria

Links to DSM–5 and ICD–10

DSM–5: Other Specified Anxiety Disorder
ICD–10: Other Specified Anxiety Disorder (F41.8)

Developing the capacities to regulate emotions, especially negative emotions, is a primary task in the first few years of life for all infants/young children. In early infancy, regulation of emotions is a dyadic process, with the infant's primary caregivers playing a primary role in helping the infant regulate and manage negative feeling states. Individual differences in infants'/young children's dispositions to certain mood states have been demonstrated, but a central role of primary caregiver relationships initially is to provide comfort for infant's distress. Through repeated experiences of being comforted, infants learn that distress can be expressed to a caregiver and relieved, and gradually over the first few years of life, young children learn to manage distress more independently as their cognitive and language skills develop.

There is ample evidence that negative emotions are more closely linked to psychopathology than positive emotions. In addition, physical expression of intense emotions is linked to reduced competence in relating to others. Two major negative mood states—depression and irritability—are ubiquitous in the experience of all individuals, including young children. When depression and irritability are not just transient feeling states but instead are severe, poorly regulated, and prolonged, they may reflect established mood disorders.

When sadness and irritability predominate in young children, especially when accompanied by vegetative symptoms (e.g., insomnia, reduced appetite, reduced activity level), Depressive Disorder of Early Childhood should be considered. However, when irritability is chronic and associated with angry and aggressive behavioral outbursts, Disorder of Dysregulated Anger and Aggression of Early Childhood should be considered. The latter represents a profound disturbance in emotional and behavioral regulation. How to best conceptualize chronic irritability and angry and aggressive outbursts has been a longstanding controversy for both older and younger children. Oppositional Defiant Disorder, Disruptive Behavior Disorder, Bipolar Disorder, and—more recently—Disruptive Mood Dysregulation Disorder all have been used to describe these patterns of dysregulation in older children. Disorder of Dysregulated Anger and Aggression of Early Childhood is an attempt to capture the salient features of these patterns in young children.

40.1 Depressive Disorder of Early Childhood

Introduction

An emerging scientific literature on early childhood mood disorders shows that young children, 3 years old and older, experience a depressive disorder that is remarkably similar to the depressive disorders presenting in later childhood and adulthood.

Developmentally sensitive modifications of the DSM–5 and ICD–10 criteria for depressive disorders include modification of the duration criteria ("more days than not for at least 2 weeks") and descriptive language that reflects how young children manifest emotional symptoms. Although depressive syndromes in infants/young children have been described in the literature since the 1930s, particularly in reaction to emotional deprivation and separation from a primary caregiver, operationalized criteria based on research for depressive syndromes in young children are emerging.

Diagnostic Algorithm

All of the following criteria must be met.

A. Depressed mood or irritability across activities, more days than not for at least 2 weeks, as indicated by either the young child's direct expression (e.g., "I'm sad") or observations made by others (e.g., the young child appears sad or is tearful, affect is flat, or the young child has frequent tantrums).

B. *Anhedonia*—which refers to markedly diminished pleasure or interest in all, or almost all, activities, such as initiation of play and interaction with caregivers—across activities, more days than not for at least 2 weeks, as indicated by either the young child's direct report or observations made by others. In young children, anhedonia may present as decreased engagement, responsivity, and reciprocity.

C. Two or more of the following must be present:

1. Significant change in appetite or failure to grow along the expected growth curve.

2. Insomnia (i.e., difficulty falling asleep or staying asleep) or hypersomnia, more days than not for at least 2 weeks.

3. Psychomotor agitation or sluggishness that is observable by others across activities, more days than not for at least 2 weeks.

4. Fatigue or loss of energy that may present as diminished exuberance across activities, more days than not for at least 2 weeks.

5. Feelings of worthlessness, excessive guilt, or self-blame in play or speech across activities, more days than not for at least 2 weeks.

6. Diminished ability to concentrate, persist, and make choices across activities, more days than not for at least 2 weeks.

7. Preoccupation with themes of death or suicide or attempts at self-harm demonstrated in speech, play, or behavior.

D. Symptoms of the disorder, or caregiver accommodations in response to the symptoms, significantly affect the young child's and family's functioning in one or more of the following ways:

1. Cause distress to the young child;

2. Interfere with the young child's relationships;

3. Limit the young child's participation in developmentally expected activities or routines;

4. Limit the family's participation in everyday activities or routines; or

5. Limit the young child's ability to learn and develop new skills or interfere with developmental progress.

Age: The diagnosis should be made with caution in young children less than 24 months old.

Duration: The symptoms must be present more days than not for at least 2 weeks.

Diagnostic Features

Depression in younger children, especially those less than 3 years old, is characterized by observable behaviors rather than the young child's direct expression of internal distress. Depressed mood and irritability that are more than transient, accompanied by vegetative symptoms or preoccupations with themes of self-harm or death, are characteristic.

Associated Features Supporting Diagnosis

Both the duration criterion for each symptom and a change in mood and behaviors must be present for a diagnosis of Depressive Disorder of Early Childhood. Young children may not be able to express their emotional distress verbally. Depressed mood may present as sad facial expression and tearfulness that are persistent, intense, and pervasive across settings and relationships. Irritability may present as temper tantrums. Potentially clinically significant tantrums are of high frequency, are pervasive across settings and relationships, and include aggression (e.g., biting, kicking, hitting). Young children with depression show greater self-harming tantrum behaviors, such as self-biting or hitting.

Anhedonia is present for more than 50% of young children with depression and is associated with greater severity of symptoms, increased family history of depression, and psychomotor retardation, suggesting that anhedonic depression in young children is similar to melancholic depression in older children and adults. Expressions of guilt, worthlessness, self-blame, and suicidal ideation need to be evaluated within a broad understanding of the young child's cognitive development. These symptoms may present in the young child's play. Disruptions in sleep, appetite, energy, and motor activity level may be more readily identified.

Although an emerging literature exists describing the neuroanatomical and neurophysiological correlates of depression in young children (which are similar to correlates at other ages), no laboratory test has yielded results of sufficient sensitivity and specificity to be used as a diagnostic tool for this disorder.

Developmental Features

In the mid-20th century, studies of infants/young children being raised in institutions led to descriptions of "anaclitic depression," which was believed to be caused by infants/young children experiencing prolonged separations from their mothers. These infants/young children experience sad facial expression, apathy, psychomotor changes and delays, failure to thrive, and lack of responsiveness to caregivers. In young children 3–5 years old, depressive symptoms are similar to those found in older children and adults with anhedonia, dysphoria, irritability, and insomnia as prominent features.

Prevalence

Prevalence rates of depression in young children 3–5 years old range from less than 0.5% to 2%.

Course

Depression in young children shows the same pattern of recurrence and persistence as depression in older children and adults. Young children with depression are much more likely to have depression in later childhood than both young children without depression and those with another mental health disorder. The strongest predictors of school-age depression are positive family affective history and early childhood depression. Note that anxiety in young children 3–5 years old also predicts school-age depression.

Risk and Prognostic Features

Young child temperament characteristics associated with early childhood depression include high negative emotionality, low emotional positivity, and behavioral inhibition. Young children of parents and grandparents with depression are at increased risk for early onset depression. Both maternal depressive symptoms and anxiety symptoms are risk factors for early onset depression. Early stressful life events mediate family history of mood disorder to increase risk for preschool onset. The young child's experience of chronic illness, multiple adverse health conditions, and pain are also associated with increased risk of early childhood depression.

Culture-Related Diagnostic Issues

Epidemiological studies in the United States and other countries have identified relatively consistent rates of early onset depression in young children. Culture-related diagnostic differences have not been identified.

Gender-Related Diagnostic Issues

The rate of early onset depression is the same for girls and boys. There is some evidence that dysregulated anger is a more prominent feature for 3- to 5-year-old boys with depression and that sadness is more prominent for young girls with depression.

Differential Diagnosis

Research has documented relationship specific depressive mood and behavioral manifestations of depression in infants/young children. It is important in young children more than 24 months old to determine whether the symptoms are manifest cross-contextually. If they are not, Relationship Specific Disorder of Infancy/Early Childhood should be considered. When depressive or irritable mood presents in young children who have experienced significant psychosocial/environmental deprivation, Reactive Attachment Disorder should be considered. Reactive Attachment Disorder is distinguished by the selective absence of attachment behaviors and the absence of vegetative symptoms. If irritability is the primary mood symptom, Disorder of Dysregulated Anger and Aggression of Early Childhood should be considered. Symptoms that help to differentiate young children with depression and tantrums from young children with Disorder of Dysregulated Anger and Aggression of Early Childhood include sleep problems, guilt, fatigue, weight changes, anhedonia, and decreased cognitive functioning. Organic diseases, such as metabolic abnormalities or space-occupying lesions, should be ruled out. Adjustment Disorder with depressive features should be considered if the onset is linked to a stressful event or circumstance. A major depressive episode that occurs in response to a psychosocial stressor is distinguished from Adjustment Disorder with depressed mood by the fact that the full criteria for a major depressive episode are not met in Adjustment Disorder.

Periods of sadness are inherent aspects of a young child's life and should not be diagnosed as a depressive episode unless criteria are met for severity, duration, and impairment.

Comorbidity

The majority of young children 3–5 years old with depression have one or more comorbid disorders, with anxiety disorders and Attention Deficit Hyperactivity Disorder among the most common comorbidities. Young children with Reactive Attachment Disorder may also have Depressive Disorder of Early Childhood. Disruptive comorbidity is very common in young children with early onset depression.

Depression often co-occurs with anxiety disorders, including phobias, and with tics. Young children with comorbid depression and anxiety may be more impaired than those with depression alone.

Links to DSM–5 and ICD–10

DSM–5: Major Depressive Disorder
ICD–10: Depressive Episode (F32)

40.2 Disorder of Dysregulated Anger and Aggression of Early Childhood

Introduction

A subset of young children struggles to develop the capacity to regulate emotions and behavior in early childhood, resulting in impairment, stigma, and exclusion from age-appropriate activities. These young children exhibit severe, frequent, and intense temper tantrums coupled with persistent irritable or angry mood. Concurrent dysregulation of emotions and behaviors has been observed and studied extensively in young children 3–5 years old, differentially conceptualized as Oppositional Defiant Disorder (ODD), comorbid mood/anxiety disorders, Disruptive Behavior Disorder, or irritability.

Disorder of Dysregulated Anger and Aggression of Early Childhood (DDAA) emerges out of research on early childhood emotional and behavioral dysregulation as well as the work on Disruptive Mood Dysregulation Disorder in older children and adults. A central component of DDAA is the focus on irritability and dysregulation of anger as expressions of emotion dysregulation that lead to dysregulated behaviors, including temper outbursts. This component of DDAA is a powerful predictor of adverse outcomes, including functional impairment and clinical diagnoses in older children.

Historically, nosologies have divided young child symptoms into either emotional or behavioral disorders. For example, ODD, included in both the DSM and ICD systems, emphasizes the young child's oppositional behaviors—including temper outburst, noncompliance, and defiance—rather than the concurrent emotion dysregulation. ICD–10 defines a "Mixed Disorder of Conduct and Emotions" (F92) that encompasses broad comorbidity between aggressive and defiant behavior and symptoms of depression, anxiety, or other emotional distress; however, this disorder does not specifically address the irritability that commonly co-occurs with ODD behaviors. Although concurrent validity and discriminant validity of ODD have been established in young children, the homotypic predictive validity of ODD (i.e., ODD in young children predicting ODD later) has been modest in most longitudinal studies. However, early childhood ODD and severe tantrums in young children have been shown to predict anxiety and mood disorders in school-age children and adolescents better than they predict Disruptive Behavior Disorder. These findings suggest that emotion dysregulation, not simply dysregulated behavior, is a critical feature of the current definition of ODD. Understanding the process as a core emotional dysregulation disorder (i.e., dysregulation of the emotion of anger and irritable affect), as defined in DDAA, has significant implications for treatment and other interventions, highlighting the importance of treating the emotional component in addition to the aggressive and disruptive behaviors.

The criteria for DDAA are derived from epidemiological studies of large cohorts of young children. Thresholds for disordered patterns are derived from rigorous assessment of these representative populations of young children using caregiver reports and observational assessments. The full distribution of symptoms in each domain is described in the criteria. The frequency and duration cut-points are empirically set to identify not more than 15% of young children, with most criteria identifying fewer than 10% to reduce the chance that typically developing young children with age-appropriate capacities for emotion regulation and behavior will be diagnosed with a disorder and to increase the chance that young children with impairments will be identified. The symptoms also must be pervasive, occurring in more than one relationship and in more than one context, and be present for at least 3 months. These specifiers allow the clinician to rule out transient, context specific, or relationship specific presentations of irritability, angry affect, and disruptive behavior.

Diagnostic Algorithm

All of the following criteria must be met.

A. The young child demonstrates a pervasive and persistent pattern of mood and behavioral dysregulation as evidenced by at least three symptoms from any of the four clusters:

1. Substantial anger and temper dysregulation demonstrated by:

    a. Has difficulty calming down when angry more days than not.

    b. Angers easily and is irritable more days than not.

    c. Shows intense or extreme temper outbursts or anger reactions more days than not.

    d. Is verbally or physically aggressive toward self or others in response to frustration or limit setting.

2. Noncompliance and rule breaking demonstrated by:

    a. Arguing with adults more days than not.

    b. Actively defying adults more days than not.

    c. Not following routine directions that the young child has the capacity to comply with, even with repeated prompts, more days than not.

    d. Breaking rules when an adult is watching at least daily.

    e. Taking things from other people or stores when it is forbidden.

3. Reactive aggression (i.e., substantial aggression when angry, upset, or scared/under threat) demonstrated by:

    a. Hits, bites, kicks, or throws things or attempts to do so at caregivers more than once a week.

    b. Hits, bites, kicks, or throws things at young children other than siblings at least once a week. (Note: For young children with limited interaction with other young children, this behavior occurs more often than not.)

    c. Breaks things on purpose at least once a week.

4. Proactive aggression demonstrated by:

    a. Often (at least once a week) is coercive and controlling in play with peers (e.g., excluding peers from play).

    b. Often (at least once a week) says things or does things that hurt other people's feelings. (Note: Only endorse if young child demonstrates understanding.)

    c. Physically or verbally frightens others.

    d. Starts physical fights.

    e. Uses or threatens to use an object to harm others.

B. Symptoms must be present in more than one setting or in more than one relationship.

C. The symptoms are not better explained by another Axis I disorder.

D. Symptoms of the disorder, or caregiver accommodations in response to the symptoms, significantly affect the young child's and family's functioning in one or more of the following ways:

1. Cause distress to the young child;

2. Cause distress to the family;

3. Interfere with the young child's relationships;

4. Limit the young child's participation in developmentally expected activities or routines;

5. Limit the family's participation in everyday activities or routines; or

6. Limit the young child's ability to learn and develop new skills or interfere with developmental progress.

Age: The young child is at least 24 months old.

Duration: The symptoms must be present for at least 3 months.

Specify:

1. Presence of limited prosocial behaviors and emotions, demonstrated by at least two of the following:
   • Patterns are present for at least 3 months
   • Lack of observable remorse or guilt
   • Lack of observable empathy for others
   • Lack of observable concern about performance

2. Aggression type: none, predominantly reactive, predominantly proactive, or combined proactive/reactive

Diagnostic Features

In DDAA, young children present with pervasive and impairing problems of both mood and behavior. DDAA incorporates four clusters of symptoms: anger, noncompliance, reactive aggression, and proactive aggression. The conceptualization of this disorder is derived from dimensional approaches in both community and clinical cohorts that characterize clinically significant emotional and behavioral dysregulation in young children. These patterns are not transient displays of challenging behaviors but rather must be present for a minimum of 3 months in more than one setting and in more than one relationship.

Associated Features Supporting the Diagnosis

Language and self-expression, self-efficacy, executive functioning, and motor activity are also developing rapidly in young children. Development in these domains may affect the development of anger regulation and behavioral regulation. For example, young children with delayed language may experience more frustration and demonstrate more signs of DDAA than young children with more advanced language development.

Developmental Features

Rates of temper tantrums and aggressive behaviors are highest in young children 3–5 years old when compared with other periods across the life span. In many outpatient early childhood clinics, these problems and hyperactivity are the most common reasons for referral. Thus, the most important developmental challenge in identifying young children with DDAA is to distinguish between typical development and disordered emotional and behavioral symptoms.

Although temper and behavioral dysregulation seen in DDAA can develop in young children less than 24 months old, the disorder cannot be diagnosed in young children until 24 months old because of the developmental capacities required to demonstrate the disorder. The consequences of poorly modulated anger and aggression are likely to increase as young children move through the early childhood years.

Prevalence

As a new disorder, the prevalence of DDAA is not established. However, because young children must demonstrate multiple criteria to meet the diagnostic criteria, the expectation is that the rate of DDAA will be significantly lower than 10%. In studies applying the criteria of disruptive mood dysregulation disorder to young children, 3%–8% of young children 3–5 years old met the full criteria. In studies of the related construct of ODD, 4%–9% of young children 2–5 years old met diagnostic criteria for the disorder. A high, stable trajectory of aggression from 17 to 42 months may be even more prevalent.

Course

No longitudinal studies of DDAA as a single entity exist, but the trajectory of symptom clusters has been examined. Young children with high levels of anger and temper dysregulation at 3 years old are at nearly twice the risk of significant depression at 6 years old compared with young children without these symptoms; furthermore, these young children are at elevated risk for anxiety, depressive patterns, and functional impairment at 9 years old. Of young children with high levels of oppositional patterns in early childhood, approximately half will continue to have high levels of oppositional patterns; moreover, as a group, they are at higher risk of internalizing and externalizing patterns of psychopathology in the school-age period. Patterns of aggression also tend to be stable. Several longitudinal studies have indicated that young children with high levels of aggression in early childhood tend to have high levels of aggression into school-age years and even into adolescence. Proactive aggression and related conduct problems are related to school-age conduct disorder as well as Attention Deficit Hyperactivity Disorder (ADHD) and defiance. In older children, proactive aggression predicts ongoing rule-breaking behaviors and eventually legal difficulties. The course of limited prosocial emotions, or callous unemotional traits, has been assessed beginning in early childhood and also shows at least moderate stability over time.

Risk and Prognostic Features

Risk factors for the signs of DDAA have been studied extensively, beginning in the prenatal period. A growing research base describes an increasingly complex set of interactions among genes and environment in the development of anger and behavioral dysregulation. In older children and adults, irritability is moderately heritable, and it is likely that early childhood irritability shares this pattern. Genes that modulate serotonin and monoamine oxidase activity have been postulated to play a role in anger-regulation problems. There is a developing literature demonstrating interactions among genetics, caregiving environment, and timing of specific exposures that influence temper and behavioral regulation.

The quality of the prenatal environment—particularly with respect to parental mental health, prenatal care, and exposure to stressors and toxins—predicts risk for DDAA. Early parenthood, in combination with other factors, such as a parental history of antisocial behaviors, has been identified as a risk factor. In the postnatal environment, exposure to coercive parenting, lack of warmth, and low family cohesion are all risk factors for DDAA. In the extreme, young child maltreatment is also a notable risk factor. There appears to be an additive effect of family socioeconomic status with other family risk factors. In particular, parental psychopathology and anger regulation are associated with higher young child dysregulation in families with low economic resources.

Young child factors related to signs of DDAA include temperamental negative affectivity and low levels of effortful control.

Positive prognostic signs include secure attachment relationships and parental sensitivity. Parenting approaches—including positive reinforcement, sensitivity, and warmth—can reduce the risk of dysregulated behavior and patterns of low prosocial behaviors or callous unemotional traits. Importantly, treatment that promotes positive parent interactions can reduce the symptoms of DDAA substantially.

Culture-Related Diagnostic Issues

The interpretation and acceptance of young child capacities for emotional and behavioral regulation take place within the values of a given cultural system. The relative values placed on autonomy, independence, and compliance influence parental and societal expectations of young children's self-regulation. Reviewing rigorous studies of older children with behavioral dysregulation suggests a striking consistency in prevalence rates of disorders across many cultures using the DSM–IV–TR nosology. This suggests that, using structured approaches, the rates of disorders of temper and behavioral regulation may be consistent across cultures, although the demarcation between typical and atypical may be defined in a culturally specific way.

Gender-Related Diagnostic Issues

Most studies of disorders of emotional and behavioral dysregulation in young children do not show a difference in rates of disorder. However, as early as the second year of life, boys show higher absolute rates of aggression and lower rates of prosocial emotional behaviors than girls. Together, these findings suggest that the impairment associated with the patterns may be different in girls and boys, potentially because of the culturally determined acceptance of the pattern.

Differential Diagnosis

The differential diagnosis of DDAA is broad. First, typical development can present with signs of DDAA, especially when families are under stress or experiencing their own symptoms of psychopathology or physical illness. Relationship specific patterns must also be differentiated from DDAA, which must present across relationships and contexts. When young children present with signs of temper dysregulation, Major Depressive Disorder should be considered, with attention to the vegetative signs of Major Depressive Disorder and anhedonia that accompany the mood symptoms. Irritability is also a possible core symptom of Generalized Anxiety Disorder, which should be ruled out. Posttraumatic Stress Disorder (PTSD) or reaction to ongoing stressors should also be considered because of the sensitivity of young children's regulation to their context. A thorough (and ongoing) social history and observations of the parent–young child relationship are necessary to assess the caregiving environment for maltreatment or suboptimal conditions that could contribute to DDAA. Insufficient sleep—because of a sleep disorder; obstructive sleep apnea; or a loud, inconsistent, or unsafe sleep environment—can present with symptoms that look like those of DDAA. Parental psychopathology or other contextual factors do not eliminate the need for diagnosing a young child's dysregulation, but, as with every disorder, provide context and may influence the development of a treatment guide.

A range of developmental processes should be considered. First, young children with limited language development may present with signs of DDAA because they have limited alternative communication strategies or because they do not understand others' language. Young children with Autism Spectrum Disorder may also present with signs of DDAA, especially when routines are disrupted, the young children experience difficulty understanding another person's experience, or in the presence of limited language. Consideration of hearing impairment is important especially when young children consistently do not follow directions. Young children with Sensory Over-Responsivity Disorder may show patterns of dysregulation related to sensory exposures.

Several prescribed pediatric medications can contribute to dysregulation. The list is extensive, but a few examples are provided here. Oral steroids, and occasionally inhaled steroids, can cause emotional, behavioral, and sleep dysregulation. Inhaled beta-adrenergic agonists, such as albuterol, can also cause periods of dysregulation that are generally not sustained. First-generation antihistamines can cause similar patterns.

Comorbidity

Most of the disorders considered in the differential diagnosis can also occur comorbidly with DDAA. For example, a young child may have comorbid ADHD and DDAA; the criteria of ADHD do not overlap directly with the criteria for DDAA. Similarly, PTSD and DDAA may co-occur but only if the signs of DDAA do not represent the reenactment signs of PTSD. Comorbidity should not be considered when all of the symptoms described in DDAA are also described in another disorder. For example, a young child should not be diagnosed with DDAA if the only DDAA symptoms are in cluster A, which could be explained by Depressive Disorder of Early Childhood.

Links to DSM–5 and ICD–10

DSM–5: Disruptive Mood Dysregulation Disorder
ICD–10: Other Persistent Mood Disorders (F34.8)

40.3 Other Mood Disorder of Early Childhood

Diagnostic Algorithm

All of the following criteria must be met.

A. The young child has one or more persistent symptoms of a mood disorder but does not meet full criteria for Depressive Disorder of Early Childhood or Disorder of Dysregulated Anger and Aggression of Early Childhood.

B. The symptoms are not already encompassed in another disorder for which the young child meets full criteria.

C. Symptoms of the disorder, or caregiver accommodations in response to the symptoms, significantly affect the young child's and family's functioning in one or more of the following ways:

1. Cause distress to the young child;

2. Interfere with the young child's relationships;

3. Limit the young child's participation in developmentally expected activities or routines;

4. Limit the family's participation in everyday activities or routines; or

5. Limit the young child's ability to learn and develop new skills or interfere with developmental progress.

Specify:

1. The disorder that best explains the young child's symptoms

2. Why the young child does not meet full criteria

Links to DSM–5 and ICD–10

DSM–5: Unspecified Depressive Disorder
ICD–10: Unspecified Mood Disorder (F39)

50 OBSESSIVE COMPULSIVE AND RELATED DISORDERS

This section encompasses Obsessive Compulsive Disorder (OCD), Tourette's Disorder, Motor or Vocal Tic Disorder, Trichotillomania, Skin Picking Disorder, and Other Obsessive Compulsive and Related Disorder. Each of these disorders is better studied and more prevalent in older children and adults, but clear evidence exists that they may present in early childhood (in some cases infancy) and be associated with impaired functioning and distress. The clinical picture in this group of disorders is perhaps more similar to the clinical picture in older children than some other groups of disorders. At least some of these disorders are genetically linked, and they also tend to cluster with anxiety disorders in some individuals.

In infants/young children, the major challenge when considering this group of diagnoses is to distinguish between individual differences within the normative range and impairing symptomatic behavior. For example, typical ritualistic behaviors and preoccupations must be distinguished from impairing obsessions and compulsions. Many infants/young children line up toys, insist on hearing the same story repeatedly, and watch the same movie again and again; however, these are not the kinds of impairing preoccupations and ritualistic compulsions that define Obsessive Compulsive Disorder. Tourette's Disorder and Motor or Vocal Tic Disorder are primarily distinguished from more transient tic disorders by the required duration of 12 months. Trichotillomania and Skin Picking Disorder are easily identified if hair pulling and skin picking are observed, but alopecia or skin lesions alone are insufficient evidence of these disorders because they may have resulted from other causes.

50.1 Obsessive Compulsive Disorder

Introduction

Obsessive Compulsive Disorder (OCD) is a severe, impairing, and often chronic disorder characterized by uncontrollable, repetitive, ritualistic thoughts and behaviors that cause distress and impairment. Although young children with early childhood-onset OCD have symptom profiles and severity that are similar to the presentation in older children, OCD in young children is not a prodromal or subthreshold version of the disorder seen at older ages. Still, it is important to assess potential obsessive and compulsive behaviors within a developmental context. It is developmentally appropriate, for example, for young children to exhibit ritualistic behaviors and insist on sameness, such as a fixed bedtime routine, and to enjoy repetitions, such as reading a book over and over again. Clinically significant obsessive and compulsive behaviors are distinguished from developmentally appropriate ritualistic and repetitive behaviors by their severity, the distress they cause the young child and the family, and the adverse impact they have on the young child's and family's functioning and the young child's development. Studies of older children have found a gap of 2 years or more between onset of OCD and diagnosis and treatment. Because effective treatment for OCD can affect the course of OCD, early identification of OCD is critical.

Diagnostic Algorithm

All of the following criteria must be met.

A. Presence of obsessions, compulsions, or both:

  1. Obsessions are evidenced by:

      a. Persistent uncontrollable preoccupation with thoughts or images that manifest as recurrent verbalizations.

  2. Compulsions are defined by:

      a. Repetitive behaviors (e.g., play enacted in a particular order, hand washing, ordering, checking, counting, repeating words silently) that the young child appears driven to perform according to rigid rules or insists that the parent perform.

      b. The young child vigorously resists or becomes markedly anxious or distressed in response to attempts to interfere with the behavior.

B. The obsessions or compulsions occur nearly every day, more days than not, and take up considerable amounts of time for the young child and parents (e.g., more than 1 hour per day).

C. The obsessions and compulsions are not attributable to another mental disorder (e.g., Trichotillomania, Atypical Eating Disorder, Autism Spectrum Disorder) medical condition (e.g., brain tumor, autoimmune process), or a substance.

D. The obsessions or compulsions are unrelated to traumatic experience.

E. Symptoms of the disorder, or caregiver accommodations in response to the symptoms, significantly affect the young child's and family's functioning in one or more of the following ways:

  1. Cause distress to the young child;

  2. Interfere with the young child's relationships;

  3. Limit the young child's participation in developmentally expected activities or routines;

  4. Limit the family's participation in everyday activities or routines;

  5. Limit the young child's ability to learn and develop new skills or interfere with developmental progress; or

  6. Result in failure to follow age-appropriate growth trajectories.

Age: The young child must be at least 36 months old.

Duration: The symptoms must be present for at least 3 months.

Specify: Whether tics are present

Note: Abrupt onset of OCD symptoms, a severe presentation, an episodic course with remission between episodes, and antecedent or concurrent infection with streptococcus or other infectious agents should prompt a comprehensive neurological and immunological evaluation.

Diagnostic Features

Young children with OCD typically present with two or more obsessions, which include contamination fears, aggressive/catastrophic obsessions, religious/scrupulosity obsessions, and somatic obsessions. Obsessions may present as intrusive thoughts that the young child expresses with repetitive questions. By definition, obsessions are distressing.

The vast majority of young children with OCD also present with multiple compulsions. The most common compulsions are washing, checking, repeating, rituals involving other people, ordering/arranging, tic-like compulsions, counting, tapping, and rubbing. Compulsions are usually linked to obsessive thoughts and are actions performed with an aim to reduce distress and anxiety.

Young children may say that they need to complete compulsions until they feel "just right" to relieve their distress. In other cases, the compulsion is performed to ward off imagined harm. However, young children often do not have the verbal capacities to express their internal states or to describe why they perform specific compulsions.

If a diagnosis of OCD is made, the clinician then specifies whether tics are present. Young children with OCD and a history of tics seem to have an earlier onset of OCD compared with young children with OCD who do not have tics.

Associated Features Supporting Diagnosis

Young children with OCD often have significant social difficulties. OCD behaviors can interfere with the young child's interactions with others and may seem bizarre. Frustration with the young child's inability to stop his or her behaviors can lead to discord with adults and with other young children. Adults often overlook or dismiss the young child's OCD behaviors. Young children also may try to hide their OCD behaviors. Both of these factors may lead to a significant gap between the onset of the illness and diagnosis and treatment.

Developmental Features

Although OCD-type behaviors are common in young children with a peak at 3 years old, they usually do not affect functioning, and they do not appear disturbingly abnormal. Potentially normative behaviors become problematic when the obsessions/compulsions are so rigid, pervasive, and distressing that they adversely affect the young child's development.

Prevalence

Estimates of the prevalence of OCD (adults, older children, and young children) range from 1% to 3%. The prevalence of early childhood onset OCD is not known, although prevalence in older children has been reported as 0.25%.

Course

The onset of early childhood OCD can be abrupt or gradual. Young children with a gradual onset appear to have the earliest onsets. The types and patterns of OCD symptoms may change over time. The course of early childhood OCD varies, although persistence of an OCD diagnosis or partial OCD symptoms is common. Some young children seem to have a chronic course, some have a waxing and waning course, and some have an episodic presentation with the young child recovering between episodes.

Risk and Prognostic Features

Family histories of OCD, tic disorder, and a non-OCD anxiety disorder are all risk factors for early childhood OCD. Stressful life events have been shown to increase OCD risk in adults and older children, although this association has not been shown for young children.

Little is known about prognostic features. Preliminary evidence suggests that girls, young children with comorbid Oppositional Defiant Disorder, and young children with greater severity of symptomatology are at increased risk for persistence of symptoms into adulthood. Also, young children with a comorbid tic disorder had higher rates of remission in later childhood and adulthood.

Culture-Related Diagnostic Issues

There are no known culture-related diagnostic issues.

Gender-Related Diagnostic Issues

Evidence for gender differences in early childhood OCD are not completely consistent. Most recent studies have found that there are no significant differences between boys and girls in the prevalence, presentation, or course of early childhood onset OCD. There also does not seem to be an association between gender and the types of disorders comorbid with OCD.

Differential Diagnosis

The first important distinction is whether the young child's OCD-type behaviors are developmentally appropriate rituals or repetitions that are calming and do not induce anxiety or distress. Differential diagnosis includes exclusion of disorders such as depression or eating disorders that may present with obsessive thoughts and disorders such as autism or cognitive delays that present with stereotypies.

An abrupt onset or worsening of OCD symptoms, antecedent or concurrent infection with streptococcus or other infectious agent, a severe presentation, and an episodic course with resolution of symptoms during episodes may be markers for Pediatric Autoimmune Neuropsychiatric Disorders Associated with a Streptococcal Infection, Pediatric Acute-onset Neuropsychiatric Syndrome, or different autoimmune encephalitides. A medical workup involving pediatric specialists in neurology, rheumatology, neuropsychiatry, and immunology should be pursued in these instances.

Comorbidity

More than 60% of young children with early childhood OCD have one or more comorbid psychiatric or developmental disorders. The most common comorbid disorders in order of prevalence are as follows: Attention Deficit Hyperactivity Disorder, tic disorders, Generalized Anxiety Disorder, Oppositional Defiant

Disorder, Specific Phobia, Separation Anxiety Disorder, Social Anxiety Disorder, and depression.

Younger age of onset for OCD has been associated with higher rates of comorbid Attention Deficit Hyperactivity Disorder and non-OCD anxiety disorders. Comorbid tics are also associated with younger age of onset.

Links to DSM–5 and ICD–10

DSM–5: Obsessive Compulsive Disorder
ICD–10: Obsessive Compulsive Disorder (F42.1)

50.2 Tourette's Disorder

Introduction

Tourette's Disorder is a tic disorder that requires the presence of both motor and phonic tics. A tic is an involuntary, repeated, rapid, nonrhythmic motor movement or vocal production that occurs suddenly and does not appear to serve any functional purpose. As young children get older, they can learn to suppress tics for varying lengths of time. Tics can be either simple, involving one movement or sound (e.g., facial grimace, throat clearing), or can involve more complex movements and sounds (e.g., shoulder shrugging followed by a head jerk, repeating sounds or words).

Diagnostic Algorithm

All of the following criteria must be met.

A. The young child demonstrates at least one simple or complex motor tic and at least one vocal tic that wax and wane in intensity.

B. The tics are not due to another medical condition.

C. Symptoms of the disorder, or caregiver accommodations in response to the symptoms, significantly affect the young child's and family's functioning in one or more of the following ways:

1. Cause distress to the young child;

2. Interfere with the young child's relationships;

3. Limit the young child's participation in developmentally expected activities or routines;

4. Limit the family's participation in everyday activities or routines; or

5. Limit the young child's ability to learn and develop new skills or interfere with developmental progress.

Age: The diagnosis should be made with caution in young children less than 18 months old.

Duration: The symptoms must be present at least 12 months.

Note: If there is an abrupt onset, consider association with streptococcal infection.

Diagnostic Features

Tourette's Disorder requires the presence of sudden, rapid, recurrent, nonrhythmic motor movements or vocalizations. Tics are considered to be involuntary and do not appear to serve any functional purpose. A young child may have different tics over time, but tics tend to recur in a similar manner with very specific timing and features. Some tics are much more common than others. For example, eye blinking, nose twitching, shoulder shrugging, throat clearing, and small whooping noises are extremely common. Young children may not be aware that they are emitting tics.

Tics can be simple movements and sounds that are quite brief, or they can be complex movements and sounds of longer duration. Complex tics may involve a series of movements and can appear purposeful, such as repetition of an obscene word (i.e., *coprolalia*) or gesture (i.e., *copropraxia*). Tics may also involve imitating movements (i.e., *echopraxia*), repeating words (i.e., *echolalia*), or repeating sounds (i.e., *palilalia*).

Tics tend to wax and wane, and there may be hours, days, or weeks in which the young child is tic-free. Persistence is established across a 12-month period, accounting for some tic-free intervals.

Associated Features Supporting Diagnosis

Young children with Tourette's Disorder often have a relative with a tic disorder or Obsessive Compulsive Disorder. Parents may not notice tics until they become more pronounced or complex.

Developmental Features

Tics tend to have similar temporal characteristics and other features through the life span, but tics may be less pronounced in young children. In addition, young children are more likely to show simple tics, which tend to emerge prior to complex tics. As young children get older, they are more likely to notice when they are emitting tics and to learn how to suppress tics for longer periods of time. As tics wax and wane, the degree of effort required to suppress tics can be highly variable. Tics generally emerge between 4 and 6 years old but can be observed as early as the second year of life.

Prevalence

Tics are common in childhood, appearing in approximately 15% of school-age children, but in most cases the tics are transient. The prevalence of Tourette's Disorder is estimated to be between 3 and 8 for every 1,000 school-age children. Prevalence in the first year of life is not known but is likely to be lower.

Course

Tics can emerge in the second year of life but more commonly are recognized as tics when young children are between 4 and 6 years old. For some young children, tics tend to worsen with age. Tics tend to emerge in a rostral/caudal manner, with facial tics emerging prior to tics involving the extremities.

Tics wax and wane in severity, and the specific muscle groups that are involved in motor and phonic tics change over time. As young children get older, they may report having a premonitory urge, or a somatic sensation of tension or needing to perform a movement, prior to expression of the tic.

Individuals may also feel a need to perform a tic in a highly particular fashion, repeating the tic until they experience a sensation of relief associated with performing the tic "just right."

Risk and Prognostic Features

Tics tend to be exacerbated by stress and fatigue. Thus, young children may exhibit more tics during periods of transition (e.g., new child care, moving to a new residence). There is strong evidence for a genetic contribution to Tourette's Disorder. In addition, obstetrical complications, lower birthweight, smoking during pregnancy, and older paternal age are associated with greater tic severity. Young children with global developmental delays and intellectual disability are at increased risk for tic disorders.

Culture-Related Diagnostic Issues

As there are cultural variations in the behaviors and sounds that are considered norm violations across cultures, a young child's tic behaviors must be evaluated in the context of his or her family's and community's cultural practices.

Gender-Related Diagnostic Issues

Tourette's Disorder is more common in boys than girls, with a gender ratio between 2:1 and 4:1.

Differential Diagnosis

Whereas tics are nonrhythmic, *motor stereotypies* are defined as rhythmic. Motor stereotypies and tics share several common features, including being involuntary, repetitive, and serving no obvious function. Commonly observed stereotypies include hand flapping, finger flicking, toe walking, and unusual body postures. It can be challenging to differentiate tics from obsessive compulsive behaviors, particularly in early childhood, when young children have difficulty reflecting on their internal experience. Grooming behaviors such as persistent hair pulling, skin picking, and nail biting appear to be more goal-directed than tics.

Comorbidity

Many young children with Tourette's Disorder have co-occurring attention and inhibitory problems or Attention Deficit Hyperactivity Disorder. Obsessive compulsive symptoms and Obsessive Compulsive Disorder are much more prevalent among young children with Tourette's Disorder and may share a common underlying etiology. Young children with Tourette's Disorder may also have difficulties with executive functioning and tasks requiring visual-motor integration.

Links to DSM–5 and ICD–10

DSM–5: Tourette's Disorder
ICD–10: Combined Vocal and Multiple Motor Tic Disorder (de la Tourette) (F95.2)

50.3 Motor or Vocal Tic Disorder

Introduction

Motor or Vocal Tic Disorder is characterized by the persistent presence of either motor or vocal tics but not both motor and vocal tics. The tics are likely to wax and wane but have been present for at least 12 months. A tic is an involuntary, repeated, rapid, nonrhythmic motor movement or vocal production that occurs suddenly and does not appear to serve any functional purpose. As young children get older, they can learn to suppress tics for varying lengths of time. Tics can be either simple, involving one movement or sound (e.g., facial grimace, throat clearing), or can involve more complex movements and sounds (e.g., shoulder shrugging followed by a head jerk or repeating sounds or words [i.e., *palilalia*]).

Diagnostic Algorithm

All of the following criteria must be met.

A. Single or multiple, simple or complex motor tics or single or multiple, simple or complex vocal tics have been present for a minimum of 12 months.

B. The tics may intensify or diminish across days and weeks, but they have been present—at least intermittently—for 12 months since the initial motor or vocal tic was observed.

C. The motor or vocal tics cannot be explained by exposure to a medication or another condition.

D. The young child does not meet criteria for Tourette's Disorder (which requires the presence of both vocal and motor tics).

E. Symptoms of the disorder, or caregiver accommodations in response to the symptoms, significantly affect the young child's and family's functioning in one or more of the following ways:

1. Cause distress to the young child;

2. Interfere with the young child's relationships;

3. Limit the young child's participation in developmentally expected activities or routines;

4. Limit the family's participation in everyday activities or routines; or

5. Limit the young child's ability to learn and develop new skills or interfere with developmental progress.

Age: The young child must be at least 36 months old.

Duration: The symptoms must be present for at least 12 months.

Specify:

1. With motor tics only

2. With vocal tics only

Links to DSM–5 and ICD–10

DSM–5: Persistent (Chronic) Motor or Vocal Tic Disorder
ICD–10: Chronic Motor or Vocal Tic Disorder (F95.1)

50.4 Trichotillomania

Introduction

Although Trichotillomania has a long history, few studies about hair pulling in infancy/early childhood have been published. Sometimes it has been considered a self-limited, benign habit. Nevertheless, several case studies have suggested that persistent and impairing hair pulling in infancy/early childhood may necessitate clinical attention.

Diagnostic Algorithm

All of the following criteria must be met.

A. The infant/young child recurrently pulls out his or her hair, resulting in areas of hair loss on the scalp, eyebrows, or eyelashes.

B. The hair loss is not attributable to a medical/dermatological condition.

C. Symptoms of the disorder, or caregiver accommodations in response to the symptoms, significantly affect the infant's/young child's and family's functioning in one or more of the following ways:

1. Cause distress to the infant/young child;

2. Interfere with the infant's/young child's relationships;

3. Limit the infant's/young child's participation in developmentally expected activities or routines;

4. Limit the family's participation in everyday activities or routines; or

5. Limit the infant's/young child's ability to learn and develop new skills or interfere with developmental progress.

Diagnostic Features

In childhood Trichotillomania, the scalp appears to be the most common site of hair pulling. Patches of alopecia are often observed. More rarely, infants/young children also pull their eyebrows and eyelashes. Recent research has begun to consistently identify two distinct hair pulling styles: "automatic" and "focused." In automatic pulling, the infant/young child does not seem aware of the pulling. In contrast, infants/young children who display focused hair pulling seem fully aware of their pulling behavior, and a frustration trigger may be detected. Finding of hair in the infant's/young child's stools is a sign that the infant/young child not only pulls but also swallows his or her hair *(trichophagia)*.

Associated Features Supporting Diagnosis

Hair pulling begins when the infant/young child is less than 3 years old; it often starts as an automatic gesture that the infant/young child performs at specific times, such as while thumb or pacifier sucking, bottle feeding, watching TV, or falling asleep. Some infants less than 12 months old pull their hair during breast-feeding. Anxious, tense, or angry family relationships have been observed as associated features in some cases.

Developmental Features

Comparisons of preschool-age and school-age children with Trichotillomania have revealed similarities and differences. Symptom severity, pleasure during pulling, and gender ratio are similar in the two age groups. Nevertheless, preschool-age children demonstrate less impairment/distress and comorbidity, pull from fewer body areas, and are less likely to be aware of the act or to report tension prior to pulling. It appears that focused hair pulling significantly increases with age, whereas automatic pulling remains consistent.

Prevalence

Because Trichotillomania is not well studied in infancy, rates of the disorder are not known.

Course

Follow-up studies of infants/young children with Trichotillomania have not been published. Among older children, studies suggest that there is an increased risk for depression and anxiety symptoms with Trichotillomania. More focused hair pulling may be associated with poorer long-term prognosis.

Risk and Prognostic Features

Family dysfunction, especially poor emotional communication, has been reported in families of infants/young children with Trichotillomania; however, it is not clear what this association means. Also, there may be a family history of Trichotillomania, Obsessive Compulsive Disorder, or anxiety disorders.

Culture-Related Diagnostic Issues

No published data are available.

Gender-Related Diagnostic Issues

There are no data regarding gender ratios of Trichotillomania among infants/young children. Among school-age children, girls tend to report greater distress and impairment associated with hair pulling, even though the frequency and severity of pulling do not seem to differ from that of boys.

Differential Diagnosis

Dermatologic conditions, such as Alopecia Areata, must be ruled out. The latter involves hair loss that is spontaneous, resulting from an auto-immune attack on hair follicles. Hair pulling is occasionally a type of stereotypy. To be considered Trichotillomania, hair pulling must result in hair loss.

Comorbidity

Trichotillomania may co-occur with anxiety disorders and depression.

Links to DSM–5 and ICD–10

DSM–5: Trichotillomania
ICD–10: Trichotillomania (F63.3)

50.5 Skin Picking Disorder of Infancy/Early Childhood

Introduction

Although skin picking is not unusual in infancy/early childhood, picking skin to the point that the infant/young child causes long-lasting wounds is unusual and concerning. The essential feature of Skin Picking Disorder is skin picking that results in long-lasting wounds.

Diagnostic Algorithm

All of the following criteria must be met.

A. The infant/young child recurrently picks at his or her skin, scabs, or minor skin anomalies, resulting in long-lasting wounds (e.g., injuries, lesions, lacerations).

B. The skin picking is not controlled by the infant/young child.

C. The lack of healing is not attributable to a medical/dermatological condition.

D. Symptoms of the disorder, or caregiver accommodations in response to the symptoms, significantly affect the infant's/young child's and family's functioning in one or more of the following ways:

1. Cause distress to the infant/young child;

2. Interfere with the infant's/young child's relationships;

3. Limit the infant's/young child's participation in developmentally expected activities or routines;

4. Limit the family's participation in everyday activities or routines; or

5. Limit the infant's/young child's ability to learn and develop new skills or interfere with developmental progress.

Diagnostic Features

The central feature of Skin Picking Disorder is persistent picking at one's own skin. Infants/young children with this disorder may pick at scabs, minor skin anomalies, or healthy skin. Sites that are most often the target of skin picking are the face, arms, hands, and legs. In addition to skin picking, some infants/young children may cause damage to their skin by rubbing, biting, or squeezing their skin.

Associated Features Supporting Diagnosis

Infants/young children may engage in a variety of rituals that precede or follow skin picking, including searching the skin and eating or playing with scabs. Some older children and adults report picking skin in response to anxiety, and others report doing so automatically, without reflecting on what they are doing.

Developmental Features

Very little is known about the developmental features of Skin Picking Disorder; the majority of cases of Skin Picking Disorder present in adolescence, and early onset cases often present to dermatologists.

Prevalence

The prevalence of skin picking in infants/young children is not known; however, in adults, approximately 1% of the population report engaging in skin picking that results in long-lasting wounds.

Course

There is very little known about the course of Skin Picking Disorder.

Risk and Prognostic Features

Skin picking tends to be exacerbated by stress. Thus, infants/young children may exhibit more skin picking during periods of transition (e.g., new child care, moving to a new residence) or other family stressors. Infants/young children with family members who have Obsessive Compulsive Disorder are at elevated risk for developing Skin Picking Disorder.

Culture-Related Diagnostic Issues

There are no known cultural variations in skin picking.

Gender-Related Diagnostic Issues

Skin Picking Disorder is more common in girls than boys.

Differential Diagnosis

Skin picking should be differentiated from insect bites that may, rarely, be a sign of neglect.

Comorbidity

Infants/young children with Skin Picking Disorder are at elevated risk for anxiety disorders, Obsessive Compulsive Disorder, Trichotillomania, and other repetitive body-focused behaviors (e.g., nail biting).

Links to DSM–5 and ICD–10

DSM–5: Excoriation (Skin-Picking) Disorder
ICD–10: Factitial Dermatitis, Neurotic Excoriation (L98.1)

50.6 Other Obsessive Compulsive and Related Disorder

Diagnostic Algorithm

All of the following criteria must be met.

A. The infant/young child has one or more persistent symptoms of Obsessive Compulsive Disorder or a related disorder but does not meet full criteria for any other disorder in this section.

B. The symptoms are not better explained by another disorder for which the infant/young child meets full criteria.

C. Symptoms of the disorder, or caregiver accommodations in response to the symptoms, significantly affect the infant's/young child's and family's functioning in one or more of the following ways:

1. Cause distress to the infant/young child;

2. Interfere with the infant's/young child's relationships;

3. Limit the infant's/young child's participation in developmentally expected activities or routines;

4. Limit the family's participation in everyday activities or routines; or

5. Limit the infant's/young child's ability to learn and develop new skills or interfere with developmental progress.

Specify:

1. The disorder that best explains the infant's/young child's symptoms

2. Why the infant/young child does not meet full criteria

Links to DSM–5 and ICD–10

DSM–5: Unspecified Obsessive Compulsive and Related Disorder
ICD–10: Obsessive Compulsive Disorder, Unspecified (F42.9)

60 SLEEP, EATING, AND CRYING DISORDERS

Disorders of sleep, eating, and excessive crying define disturbances in basic physiological activities necessary for healthy development and even survival. Sleep, feeding, and crying are behaviors that are ubiquitous, and disturbances in them may be the result of many other disorders. The disorders defined in this section are intended to define disturbances that are primary rather than symptoms of other disorders.

Compared with many other early childhood disorders, disorders of sleep, eating, and excessive crying are more likely to present in the first year of life and more likely to be encountered in primary care settings. Problems in sleeping, eating, and crying are quite common in infants/young children, and perturbations within the normative range in these domains are not considered clinical abnormalities. Disorders in this section—defined by disturbed sleep or eating, or by excessive crying—must impair the functioning of the infant/young child, the family, or both.

Although these disorders are defined in terms of infant/young child behaviors and are considered disorders existing within an individual infant/young child, they are each closely linked to instrumental caregiving tasks because of the dependency of infants/young children on caregivers for survival. Differences in caregivers' tolerances for sleep, eating, and crying are well documented, and cultural beliefs define parameters of how individual differences are understood and responded to. Sleep, eating, and crying also undergo significant changes from the first year of life through the preschool years. Because of the inextricable links among caregiving and infant/young child sleep, eating, and crying, careful attention to the question of relationship specificity is important, especially for sleep and eating. Unless there is clear evidence of the symptomatic behavior being limited to the context of a specific relationship, a sleep disorder, eating disorder, or crying disorder should be identified.

Sleep Disorders

Introduction

Sleep problems are among the most common concerns in early childhood. Sleep patterns change dramatically over the course of the first 5 years of life, and there is substantial variability across individual infants/young children. Among early childhood mental health problems, sleep disorders may have the most profound direct influence on sleep in other family members, often with reciprocal influences between the infant's/young child's and parents' sleep. Although sleep patterns develop in the caregiving context, sleep problems reflect the interactions of biology, caregiving relationships, and physical sleep environment. Research and clinical experience indicate that significant sleep problems can develop in the context of healthy relationships as well as within higher risk contexts.

Sleep patterns evolve substantially in the first years of life, but the majority of typically developing infants are able to sleep through the night by 6 months, and it is possible for sleep problems to cause severe impairment and distress in the second half of the first year of life.

Much of what we know about sleep in infants/young children is from broadly defined parent reports of sleep problems, resulting in a literature that has more frequently examined correlates and course of sleep problems than specific disorders. In addition, much of what we know is likely culture bound, and clinicians are cautioned about applying norms about sleep behavior in cultures from which the norms have not been derived.

This section includes four disorders: Sleep Onset Disorder, Night Waking Disorder, Partial Arousal Sleep Disorder, and Nightmare Disorder of Early Childhood. The disorders are defined empirically on the basis of existing knowledge about typical sleep and require impairment to ensure that nonpathological patterns are not considered disorders.

Consistent with the DC:0–5 approach to early childhood mental health problems, sleep disorders do not ascribe etiology to the problem. However, it is clear that sleep patterns develop in the family context, dependent on family decisions about where to sleep, the sleep context and routines, and family responses to the infant's/young child's signaling. The evolution of sleep patterns in the first few years represents a complex interaction of cultural expectations, physical conditions and socioeconomic factors, family stressors and resilience, parenting factors, infant's/young child's own intrinsic factors, and the interaction among these factors.

60.1 Sleep Onset Disorder

Diagnostic Algorithm

All of the following criteria must be met.

A. The infant/young child requires more than 30 minutes to fall asleep most nights in a week.

B. The sleep problem is not better explained by a symptom of another disorder.

C. Symptoms of the disorder, or caregiver accommodations in response to the symptoms, significantly affect the infant's/young child's and family's functioning in one or more of the following ways:

1. Cause distress to the infant/young child;

2. Interfere with the infant's/young child's relationships;

3. Limit the infant's/young child's participation in developmentally expected activities or routines;

4. Limit the family's participation in everyday activities or routines; or

5. Limit the infant's/young child's ability to learn and develop new skills or interfere with developmental progress.

Age: The infant/young child must be at least 6 months old.

Duration: The symptoms must be present for at least 4 weeks.

Links to DSM–5 and ICD–10

DSM–5: Insomnia Disorder
ICD–10: Nonorganic Insomnia (F51.0)

60.2 Night Waking Disorder

Diagnostic Algorithm

All of the following criteria must be met.

A. Multiple or prolonged awakenings, accompanied by signaling, most nights of the week.

B. Symptoms are not better explained by other disorders or medical problems and medication side effects.

C. Symptoms of the disorder, or caregiver accommodations in response to the symptoms, significantly affect the infant's/young child's and family's functioning in one or more of the following ways:

1. Cause distress to the infant/young child;

2. Interfere with the infant's/young child's relationships;

3. Limit the infant's/young child's participation in developmentally expect-ed activities or routines;

4. Limit the family's participation in everyday activities or routines; or

5. Limit the infant's/young child's ability to learn and develop new skills or interfere with developmental progress.

Age: The infant/young child is at least 8 months old.

Duration: The symptoms must be present for at least 4 weeks.

Links to DSM–5 and ICD–10

DSM–5: Insomnia Disorder
ICD–10: Nonorganic Insomnia (F51.0)

60.3 Partial Arousal Sleep Disorder

Diagnostic Algorithm

Of the following criteria, either A or B must be met, and both C and D must be met.

A. Sleep terrors: Frequent, recurrent episodes of sudden arousals from sleep, although not to a fully awakened state. The episodes often are associated with screaming and signs of distress, including palpitations, increased respiratory rate, and diaphoresis. These events usually occur within the first few hours of sleep. In a sleep terror, young children do not readily respond to efforts to arouse them during these events.

or

B. Sleep walking: Frequent, recurrent episodes of arising from bed and walking around the home. During episodes, the young child has open eyes but has lim-ited responsiveness.

C. The young child has no discernable recollection of the event in the morning.

D. Symptoms of the disorder, or caregiver accommodations in response to the symptoms, significantly affect the young child's and family's functioning in one or more of the following ways:

1. Cause distress to the young child;

2. Interfere with the young child's relationships;

3. Limit the young child's participation in developmentally expected activi-ties or routines;

4. Limit the family's participation in everyday activities or routines; or

5. Limit the young child's ability to learn and develop new skills or interfere with developmental progress.

Age: The young child is at least 12 months old.

Duration: The symptoms should be present for at least 1 month.

Links to DSM–5 and ICD–10

DSM–5: Non-Rapid Eye Movement Sleep Arousal Disorder—Sleep Terror Type
ICD–10: Sleep Terrors (F51.4)

60.4 Nightmare Disorder of Early Childhood

Diagnostic Algorithm

All of the following criteria must be met.

A. Repeated occurrence of bad dreams or sudden awakenings with distress that occur most often in the second half of the sleep period. The young child may or may not recall or report content.

B. The dreams do not occur solely as a result of Posttraumatic Stress Disorder or Separation Anxiety Disorder.

C. Symptoms of the disorder, or caregiver accommodations in response to the symptoms, significantly affect the young child's and family's functioning in one or more of the following ways:

    1. Cause distress to the young child;

    2. Interfere with the young child's relationships;

    3. Limit the young child's participation in developmentally expected activities or routines;

    4. Limit the family's participation in everyday activities or routines; or

    5. Limit the young child's ability to learn and develop new skills or interfere with developmental progress.

Age: The young child is at least 12 months old.

Duration: The symptoms should be present for at least 1 month.

Links to DSM–5 and ICD–10

DSM–5: Nightmare Disorder
ICD–10: Nightmares (F51.5)

Note: The following sections apply to all Sleep Disorders.

Diagnostic Features

The essential feature of any sleep disorder in infants/young children is a pattern of insufficiently initiated or maintained nighttime sleep behavior that is culturally nonnormative, sustained for at least 1 month, and functionally impairing.

The impairment associated with sleep problems is important to highlight because of the broad range of typical sleep patterns over the first 5 years of life, including in the latter half of the first year of life. An infant/young child who meets frequency or duration criteria for any sleep disorder but who does not meet the impairment criteria does not have a sleep disorder. Impairment may present as internalizing or externalizing patterns, and impairment related to sleep disorders can be seen in both the infant/young child and the caregiver. Sleep deprivation in infants/young children may present with distractibility, irritability, or a need for additional daytime sleep. Parents who are sleep deprived may be tired, may feel overextended, and may similarly experience impaired cognition and negative mood patterns.

Associated Features Supporting Diagnosis

Sleep disorders in general, and night awakenings and nightmares in particular, are associated with internalizing and externalizing patterns in infants/young children. The causal direction of associations may be bidirectional or unidirectional. Separation anxiety has been specifically associated with night awakenings, nightmares, and sleep waking. Externalizing patterns and hyperactivity and impulsivity have also been associated night awakenings. Interestingly, sleep efficiency has also been associated with measures of emotional knowledge and narrative coherence in attachment assessments.

Developmental Features

To identify abnormal sleep behavior, it is necessary to recognize the developmental process and range of typical sleep patterns in the first 5 years of life. The first 12 months of life are a period of sleep consolidation that contains the most dramatic change in sleep patterns. At birth, infants wake every 2–3 hours at night. Initially, they tend to be more alert at night and to sleep more during the day. Approximately half of infants will be able to sleep through the night by 4 months, when the capacity to self-soothe begins to develop. By 12 months old, 85% of infants sleep 8–9 hours overnight.

Although there is tremendous variability across individual sleep patterns, sleep onset latency in infants/young children is greater than 30 minutes in a small proportion of infants/young children. Variability in sleep onset latency may be influenced by sleep association patterns in infants/young children more than 4 months old, meaning that they may depend on specific routines, transitional objects, or people present to fall asleep. In young children, parental limit setting may also play a role in the sleep onset delay.

In terms of night awakenings, according to research in North America, about one half of infants sleep through the night by 8 weeks, and 75% of infants sleep through the night by 12 months.

Nightmares and partial arousals do not develop until later in toddlerhood and are highest in the preschool years. Developmentally, it is important to note that many young children may not remember the content of their dreams. Compared with adults, nightmares in young children can happen more commonly without an identified traumatic exposure, although the social context is important to consider clinically.

Prevalence

Prevalence of Sleep Onset Disorder is somewhat difficult to assess because of variability of criteria used in epidemiologic studies. Approximately 10%–15% of infants/young children have a sleep onset latency of greater than 30 minutes by parent report. When using rigorous criteria that include impairment, rates of sleep disorders are 5%–10% in U.S. and European studies, but as many as one third of parents report sleep problems using more general terminology, with higher rates in the second half of the first year of life.

Nightmares and partial arousals are categorized as parasomnias, which occur commonly in the preschool-age group. Only about 1%–3% of young children experience nightmares in a frequency of "often" or more, but many more young children have occasional nightmares.

Course

Sleep problems in infancy are not highly predictive of later sleep problems in the preschool-age group. Approximately 30%–40% of infants 8–10 months old continue to have a sleep problem reported by a parent in the preschool years. Overall, unlike most early childhood mental health problems, young children show variability in sleep patterns over time. The exception to this pattern is nightmares, which show higher rates of stability from 24 to 60 months.

Early sleep dysregulation has been posited to be associated with later adverse outcomes, including language development. Sleep problems in the first 42 months of life, resulting in overall less sleep, have been shown to be associated with hyperactivity problems at 6 years old. Similarly, early sleep problems predict poorer cognitive outcomes, including lower language scores and spatial reasoning. Insufficient sleep in the first 3 years of life predicts higher rates of obesity at 6 years old. Importantly, short sleep duration at 18 months is a strong predictor of hyperactivity at 60 months.

Risk and Prognostic Features

Infant/young child biological factors as well as family factors are associated with risk of sleep problems. Heritability of sleep problems, including night terrors, is high. Infants/young children with sleep problems are more likely to have a difficult temperament and to be difficult to soothe. In addition, medical problems such as gastroesophageal reflux and neurodevelopmental disorders are also associated with a higher risk of sleep difficulties.

Research suggests that infants/children with more sleep difficulties, especially sleep onset problems and nighttime awakenings, may have atypical diurnal cortisol patterns, particularly higher morning cortisol or mean cortisol levels. Whether this association indicates a biological risk factor or sequellae of sleep deprivation is not established.

Family factors associated with sleep problems in early childhood include mental health issues, parents' sleep-related behaviors, and cognitions. Infants born to mothers with depression in pregnancy are at higher risk for sleep problems, even when controlling for postpartum maternal symptoms. Postnatal parental depression, primarily studied in mothers, and parental sleep problems have been shown to be associated with infant/young child sleep problems, although the direction of this association is difficult to establish. Sleep difficulties are associated with parenting behaviors surrounding sleep, although this association is most likely transactional rather than unidirectional. Infants whose parents are actively involved in falling asleep—through holding, feeding, or rocking—are at higher risk of sleep disorders than infants who fall asleep in their crib with minimal parental assistance. After 5 months old, when nighttime awakenings are unlikely to indicate hunger, infants who are fed with nocturnal arousals are also more likely to have more difficulties with falling asleep. Daytime use of physical contact to calm an infant is associated with more sleep problems. Parental cognitions that indicate difficulty with limit setting and anger at an infant's needs also predict infant sleep problems, as do beliefs that an infant needs immediate response to reduce distress during sleep and maternal separation anxiety. These associations between cognitions and sleep problems are mediated by parental behaviors.

Other factors, including socioeconomic status and family structure, do not appear to independently influence the risk of sleep problems, except as they influence parenting behaviors related to sleep.

Culture-Related Diagnostic Issues

Sleep expectations are culturally defined; therefore, disorders must be considered in the cultural context in which they occur. In most of the world, infants sleep with their parents, sharing a bed. Research indicates that co-sleeping in and of itself is not associated with sleep problems. Few studies have examined variability of presentation of sleep concerns in the first years of life. In Asian countries, parents report higher rates of sleep problems and reduced sleep duration compared with parents from predominantly English-speaking countries. Whether these differences represent culture or biology is not clear, and it is most important to note that the variability within each group was as broad as the differences between the groups.

Gender-Related Diagnostic Issues

There are no consistent data suggesting a gender difference in sleep problems or infant signaling. Boys may be at higher risk of restless sleep than girls.

Differential Diagnosis

Differential diagnosis of sleep problems in infancy/early childhood is limited. First, perceived sleep problems must be distinguished from typical sleep patterns or developmentally inappropriate expectations. The context of sleep—including schedule, noises in or around the home, and the parents' sleep schedule (especially parents who work at nights or return home during the night)—should be assessed. Excessive daytime sleep may also influence nighttime sleep patterns, resulting in delayed sleep onset or early awakenings. It is important to differentiate typical patterns from disorders that require intervention and support, indicating infant/young child or parental sleep deprivation or irritability.

If there is evidence that an infant's/young child's sleep is consistently aberrant in one setting (e.g., with parents) and is consistently not aberrant in another setting (e.g., grandparents), Relationship Specific Disorder of Infancy/Early Childhood (sleep) is the appropriate diagnosis. In the absence of clear evidence of variability in different contexts (e.g., the infant/young child only sleeps at home at nighttime), a sleep disorder should be diagnosed. Variability between daytime naps and nighttime sleep should not be considered variability in different contexts for this purpose.

Posttraumatic Stress Disorder should be considered in infants/young children presenting with nightmares or bad dreams, which occur more commonly in infants/young children exposed to traumatic events than those who have not experienced traumatic events.

Separation Anxiety Disorder should be considered in infants/young children who have delayed sleep onset when sleeping alone but not when co-sleeping.

Medications or other agents can also interfere with sleep. Caffeine, steroids, and some cold and cough agents are of particular note. So-called paradoxical effects can be seen in some young children taking antihistamines, resulting in increased agitation instead of the commonly described sedation.

Breathing-related sleep problems, such as apnea, may also present as frequent arousals, although they call for a different intervention. These infants/young children also have audible snoring and may have brief periods of apnea (not breathing) often followed by a jagged sounding catch-up breath or snore. When unclear, a pediatric sleep study may be a helpful tool to identify underlying sleep patterns or troubles.

A broad differential diagnosis should be considered in the case of acute onset, rather than chronic, sleep problems, which may reflect a medical problem, a response to a stressful life event, or changes in the sleep environment.

Comorbidity

In Sleep Onset Disorder, nocturnal awakenings are commonly associated with emotional and behavioral disturbances, including most anxiety disorders, mood disorders, and Attention Deficit Hyperactivity Disorder. This association may operate in either direction as sleep deprivation exacerbates dysregulation and anxiety, while disruptive behavior and internalizing symptoms can contribute to sleep dysregulation.

Eating Disorders of Infancy/Early Childhood

Introduction

Eating disorders in infants/young children are among the most common behavioral disturbances that lead parents to seek treatment in primary care settings. Some 25%–40% of infants/young children are reported by their caregivers to have feeding problems—mainly slow feeding, refusal to eat, picky eating, or vomiting.

The various eating disorders are defined descriptively by observable symptomatic behaviors that manifest cross-contextually rather than by inferred etiologies. In a given case, of course, contributors to the behavioral patterns may be made to direct appropriate treatment, but the extant evidence does not permit linking eating patterns with specific etiologies in most cases. Sensory aversions, regulation problems, and fearful behaviors from exposure to traumatic medical procedures to the mouth and throat all have been implicated in eating problems and can be noted as associated features that are important for treatment planning. In addition, caregivers' interactions during feeding may be responsive, controlling, indulgent, or neglectful. An infant's/young child's interactions may be cooperative, resistant (e.g., turning the head away from food), or conflicted (e.g., throwing food). These behaviors also may be useful to note. Medical conditions associated with the eating disorder should be noted under Axis III.

60.5 Overeating Disorder

Diagnostic Algorithm

All of the following criteria must be met.

A. Young children with this disorder overeat or attempt to overeat by demonstrating each of the following:

1. The young child persistently seeks excessive amounts of food during meals/feedings.

2. The young child repeatedly seeks or eats excessive amounts of food between mealtimes or scheduled feedings.

B. Young children with this disorder are excessively preoccupied with food and eating, as manifest by at least two of the following:

1. The young child takes food from others or forages from garbage bins.

2. The young child stuffs food in the cheeks when eating.

3. The young child talks repeatedly about food (e.g., the next meal) or food themes predominate in the infant/young child's play.

C. The young child becomes distressed if prevented from engaging in the behaviors in criterion A.

D. The young child's behavior is not due to a condition that better accounts for the behaviors (e.g., food unavailability and hunger, medication side effects, or medical conditions).

E. Symptoms of the disorder, or caregiver accommodations in response to the symptoms, significantly affect the young child's and/or family's functioning in one or more of the following ways:

1. Cause distress to the young child;

2. Interfere with the young child's relationships;

3. Limit the young child's participation in developmentally expected activities or routines;

4. Limit the family's participation in everyday activities or routines;

5. Limit the young child's ability to learn and develop new skills, or interfere with developmental progress; or

6. Result in failure to follow age-appropriate growth trajectories.

Age: The diagnosis is not made in children less than 24 months old.

Duration: The symptoms must be present for more than 1 month.

Specify: If the young child's weight is above the 95th percentile, this is noted under Axis III.

Diagnostic Features

The young child's overconsumption or attempted overconsumption of food, as well as search for and preoccupation with food, are pervasive symptoms rather than transient anomalies. Furthermore, they are pervasive in that they are evident beyond any specific relational context. If the behaviors are limited to a specific relational context, the diagnosis of Relationship Specific Disorder of Infancy/Early Childhood with manifestations of overeating/overfeeding behaviors is appropriate.

Associated Features Supporting Diagnosis

The main clinical feature of this disorder is the young child's preoccupation with food, at the expense of other developmentally appropriate activities. The young child becomes distressed if prevented from engaging in these behaviors and may have nonspecific symptoms of anxiety, irritability, or anger.

Developmental Features

Overeating Disorder is rarely seen in young children less than 2 years old, because some degree of autonomy as well as verbal and motor skills are required to search for the food. Overfeeding occurs in young children less than 2 years old, especially during the first year of life. If there are no other behaviors indicating search for and preoccupation with food, then criteria for the disorder will not be met.

Prevalence

Data on the prevalence of Overeating Disorder in the first years of life are limited. In community studies, excessive appetite is reported for 10% of young children. Awareness of the potentially pathological significance of overeating has been lower than for Undereating Disorder.

Course

There are no systematic studies about the course of the disorder. Clinical experience suggests that the behaviors tend to be persistent and may be unlikely to remit spontaneously. The relationship between overeating in early childhood and Binge Eating or Bulimia Nervosa at later ages is unknown.

Risk and Prognostic Features

Risk factors for obesity include genetic predisposition, feeding patterns and diet early in life, reduced physical activity, medication use, and other exposures. In addition, food marketing and promotion and accessibility to healthy or unhealthy food may contribute to overeating.

A chronic mismatch of caregiver responsiveness to young child feeding cues, such as feeding when the young child is not hungry, has been shown to have a role in the development of overeating by impairing the young child's response to internal states of hunger and satiation. Caregivers' exerting excessive control over what and how much young children eat also may contribute to childhood overeating.

Caregiver eating disorders—including Binge Eating, Bulimia Nervosa, and Anorexia Nervosa—may increase risk factors for all types of eating disorders in young children, including overeating. Maternal symptoms of stress, depression, and anxiety have been related to nonresponsive feeding styles (e.g., controlling, indulgent, uninvolved). Nonresponsive feeding, in turn, has been related to under- or overweight conditions among young children. Family conflicts around food are quite commonly associated with eating disorders in young children.

Culture-Related Diagnostic Issues

No data exist about culture-related diagnostic issues, although one may assume that different cultures have different norms of what is the optimal and healthy eating pattern. For instance, Western societies strongly reinforce "values" of thinness and "healthy" foods, whereas in developing countries where resources are scarce, the emphasis is on survival.

Gender-Related Diagnostic Issues

No specific data are available regarding gender differences.

Differential Diagnosis

Medical conditions such as Prader-Willi syndrome and hypothyroidism should be considered. Medication side effects should also be considered.

Comorbidity

Although data are limited, comorbid diagnoses of Sensory Processing Disorder and Depressive Disorder of Early Childhood may co-occur with Overeating Disorder.

Links to DSM–5 and ICD–10

DSM–5: Unspecified Feeding or Eating Disorder
ICD–10: Overeating Associated With Other Psychological Disturbances (F50.4)

60.6 Undereating Disorder

Diagnostic Algorithm

All of the following criteria must be met.

A. The infant/young child consistently eats less than expected for his or her age.

B. The infant/young child exhibits one or more of the following maladaptive eating behaviors:

1. Consistent lack of interest in eating.

2. Fearful avoidance of eating.

3. Difficulty regulating state during feedings (e.g., repeatedly falls asleep or becomes agitated).

4. Eating only while asleep.

5. Failure to transition to solid foods.

6. Eating only when specific conditions imposed by him or her are fulfilled by caregivers (e.g., in front of television with a specific program, with toys and stories).

7. Extremely picky and selective, refuses to eat certain colors or textures of food or unusually restricted range of foods.

8. Pouching (prolonged maintenance of food in mouth without swallowing).

C. The maladaptive eating behavior is not better explained by a medical condition or medication side effect.

D. Symptoms of the disorder, or caregiver accommodations in response to the symptoms, significantly affect the infant's/young child's and family's functioning in one or more of the following ways:

1. Cause distress to the infant/young child;

2. Interfere with the infant's/young child's relationships;

3. Limit the infant's/young child's participation in developmentally expected activities or routines;

4. Limit the family's participation in everyday activities or routines;

5. Limit the infant's/young child's ability to learn and develop new skills or interfere with developmental progress; or

6. Result in failure to follow age-appropriate growth trajectories.

Age: There are no age specifications.

Duration: The symptoms must be present for more than 1 month.

Specify:

1. Whether there is weight loss

2. Whether there is lack of expected weight gain

Note: Weight loss or lack of expected weight gain due to undereating should be noted under Axis III.

Diagnostic Features

The main eating behaviors that bring the infant/young child to the clinician's attention include refusal to eat solids, poor appetite, selective eating, and fear of choking. Weight loss or lack of expected weight gain is clearly possible but is not a necessary criterion because some infants/young children do have pathological patterns of eating but maintain weight. For instance, some infants/young children refuse to eat solids but drink several bottles per day.

Associated Features Supporting Diagnosis

Prolonged mealtimes, stressful mealtimes, lack of appropriate autonomous feeding, nocturnal eating (after 1 year old), prolonged breast- or bottle-feeding, and failure to taste new textures are common associated features.

Picky eating is not necessarily associated with low weight, although it is often associated with tension and distress in the families of these infants/young children. Some infants/young children may exhibit aversion to specific smells, textures, and tastes.

Developmental Features

Undereating may appear in the earliest months of life. Sometimes this may be relationship specific undereating, in which case Relationship Specific Disorder of Infancy/Early Childhood is the appropriate diagnosis. If the undereating occurs in more than one relationship, Undereating Disorder should be considered and may be associated with being underfed. In the first year of life, feeding begins as a dyadic activity. In the latter part of the first year, infants gradually begin to feed themselves—initially, these efforts are limited, but eating becomes increasingly more independent during the second and third years of life. Selective picky eating may appear in the second half of the first year, especially at the transition to solid foods. Some infants may resist weaning from breastfeeding. Still, selective eating may start at any age.

Prevalence

Some 25%–40% of infants/young children are reported by their caregivers to have feeding problems—mainly vomiting, slow feeding, and refusal to eat. Although some of these difficulties are transient, some problems, such as refusal to eat, are found in 3%–10% of infants/young children and tend to persist.

Course

The available prospective research suggests some degree of continuity of eating problems from infancy to older ages, including adolescence and adulthood. For example, some 40% of the irregular eaters at 5 years old were still irregular eaters at 14 years old. Independent contributions include the infants'/young children's own capacity to regulate their sleep and mood as well as the infant's/young child's relationship with caregivers during the early years. Infants with severe eating disorders tend to exhibit more subsequent emotional and behavioral problems than controls but not necessarily more eating problems. Many of the outcome studies consider eating and sleeping disorders in infancy to be symptoms of physiological dysregulation and combine the data on eating, sleeping, and other dysregulated behavior. Infants/young children with crying, sleeping, or eating problems have more behavioral problems than controls, especially in multiproblem families. Selective (picky) eating often improves spontaneously over time, especially when parents stop reacting to the infant's/young child's eating behavior (e.g., either praising or criticizing). Other infants/young children maintain picky eating behavior into adulthood. Long-term outcome studies of infants/young children with Undereating Disorder are still lacking.

Risk and Prognostic Features

Maternal eating disturbances, including Bulimia Nervosa and Anorexia Nervosa, are a risk factor for all types of eating disorders in infancy. Maternal symptoms of stress, depression, and anxiety have been related to nonresponsive feeding styles (e.g., controlling, indulgent, uninvolved). Nonresponsive feeding, in turn, has related to under- or overweight conditions among infants/young children. Family conflicts around food are common, and the tension becomes a risk factor in itself for aggravation of the eating problem. Picky eating is often observed in parents of picky-eating infants/young children.

Culture-Related Diagnostic Issues

Eating plays an important role in most cultures, acceptable eating habits vary widely between religious and ethnic groups, and eating disorders have been conceptualized as culture-bound syndromes. In this context, it is notable that most published research addresses North American and European populations.

Gender-Related Diagnostic Issues

There are no published data about the gender distribution of Undereating Disorder in infancy. Although there are gender differences in eating disorders later in childhood/adolescence/adulthood (with females more likely to experience eating disorders), no gender differences have been noted in eating disorders in infancy and early childhood.

Differential Diagnosis

Given the reliance of infants/young children on caregivers, eating is a dyadic process. The term *feeding* reflects the adult's role in the process, whereas the term *eating* reflects the infant's/young child's role (e.g., opening the mouth, swallowing, reaching for the food). Feeding practices of parents have been found to be strongly associated with both infants'/young children's over- and undereating behaviors. This finding raises the question of whether problematic feeding interactions are relational or within-the-infant/young-child disorders. As a rule, unless there is evidence that the infant's/young child's eating problems are limited to one or more primary caregivers, the diagnosis is an eating disorder. If there is evidence that the infant/young child undereats or overeats only with one caregiver, the diagnosis would be Relationship Specific Disorder of Infancy/Early Childhood, with a specification of eating disturbance.

One needs to rule out organic reasons for Undereating Disorder, such as a milk allergy; structural abnormalities that affect the naso-oropharynx, the larynx and trachea, and the esophagus; neurodevelopmental disabilities; oral hypersensitivity and oral-motor dysfunction; systemic illnesses; as well as organic causes of pain, such as esophagitis due to gastroesophageal reflux.

Comorbidity

Coexisting medical problems should be mentioned under Axis III because good medical management does not always alleviate feeding problems adequately. For instance, young children with cystic fibrosis often have a pattern of eating slowly, chewing with difficulty, preferring liquids, refusing to eat solids, and being averse to new food. Infants with gastroesophageal reflux have lower intake of energy-generating food, have fewer adaptive skills and less readiness for solids, are more likely to refuse food, and are more demanding and difficult at feeding time. Relationship Specific Disorder of Infancy/Early Childhood with manifestations other than eating problematic behaviors may co-occur with the diagnosis of Undereating Disorder.

Links to DSM–5 and ICD–10

DSM–5: Unspecified Feeding or Eating Disorder
ICD–10: Other Eating Disorders (F50.8)

60.7 Atypical Eating Disorder

Diagnostic Algorithm

All of the following criteria must be met.

A. The infant/young child exhibits abnormal eating symptoms that include at least one of the following:

1. *Hoarding*—the infant/young child hides food in unusual places (e.g., in the bed, in a desk drawer).

2. *Pica*—habitual eating of nonnutritive substances.

3. *Rumination*—a pattern of regurgitating and reswallowing food.

B. The infant's/young child's abnormal eating behavior is not better explained by a medical condition or medication side effect.

C. Symptoms of the disorder, or caregiver accommodations in response to the symptoms, significantly affect the infant's/young child's and family's functioning in one or more of the following ways:

1. Cause distress to the infant/young child;

2. Interfere with the infant's/young child's relationships;

3. Limit the infant's/young child's participation in developmentally expected activities or routines;

4. Limit the family's participation in everyday activities or routines;

5. Limit the infant's/young child's ability to learn and develop new skills or interfere with developmental progress; or

6. Result in failure to follow age-appropriate growth trajectories.

Age: There are no age specifications.

Duration: The symptoms must be present for 1 month.

Specify:

1. Which atypical eating pattern is present

Note: Medical complications, such as dental caries or anemia resulting from atypical eating behaviors, should be noted under Axis III.

Diagnostic Features

Atypical Eating Disorder symptoms are heterogeneous in presentation. For all three types of atypical eating symptoms, diagnostic criteria for the disorder are met only if the young child's abnormal eating behavior is pervasive across all contexts and associated with impaired functioning.

Hoarding describes a pattern of hiding/storing food in unusual places, even though it may not be eaten. It must be distinguished from children who hide food they do not like so that they do not have to eat it. Hoarding is more pervasive and not limited to undesired foods.

Pica describes persistent eating of nonfood substances, such as dirt, chalk, paper, soap, cloth, string, wool, soil, paint, gum, hair, ice, clay, starch, metal or plastic objects, or feces. Pica is usually not associated with general aversion to food. These objects are not eaten in lieu of food but in addition to food.

Rumination describes the repeated regurgitation of food that follows feeding or eating. Usually the infant/young child reswallows the regurgitated food, but sometimes the food is expelled following regurgitation.

Associated Features Supporting Diagnosis

Hoarding: Finding food in unusual places helps to make the diagnosis. Some of these young children are overweight, whereas some are underweight, depending on what they do with the hidden food. Hoarding has been associated with young child maltreatment, especially neglect.

Pica: Iron and zinc deficiencies have been reported in some cases of pica. Some cases of pica are diagnosed following intestinal obstruction or perforation; infections such as toxoplasmosis and toxocariasis following ingestion of feces, soil or dirt; and lead poisoning. Pica has sometimes been associated with intellectual disabilities, autism, and other developmental disabilities.

Rumination: During rumination, an infant often arches his or her back with the head held back, while making sucking movements with the tongue, and seems to be engaged in a self-soothing or self-stimulating activity. Between meals, the infant may be hungry and irritable. Weight loss and failure to gain weight are common, up to the point of malnutrition, especially when the regurgitation follows every meal.

Developmental Features

Hoarding: To our best knowledge, hoarding has not been described in young children less than 2 years old.

Pica: In young children less than 2 years old, developmentally normal mouthing of objects may result in ingestion; therefore, there is a need to be cautious when giving the diagnosis of pica in young children less than 24 months old.

Rumination: Rumination can be observed across the age range, from infancy to adulthood. In infants, it usually starts between 3 and 12 months.

Prevalence

The prevalence of hoarding, pica, and rumination in young children is unknown. Picky eating is much more common, although the exact figures in the general population are unknown.

Course

Hoarding: There are no published data on its course over time, although clinical experience suggests that it often resolves within weeks to months of the young child being placed in an adequate caregiving environment.

Pica can occur in otherwise typically developed young children, although the phenomenon is more common in young children with diagnoses of intellectual disability and autism. The course of the disorder depends on its severity and may become protracted and lead to medical emergencies.

Rumination may be self-limited, but it may also become protracted, leading to potentially fatal malnutrition. Some cases have an episodic course; other cases are continuous.

Risk and Prognostic Features

Pica: The main risk factors are significant developmental delay, lack of parental supervision, and neglect. The prognosis for pica is related to the presence of these factors in addition to the potential medical complications of the ingestion of nonfood materials.

Rumination and *Hoarding:* Environmental risk factors include neglect, lack of stimulation, and severely disordered parent–infant/young child relationships.

Culture-Related Diagnostic Issues

Pica: In some cultures, ingestion of soil is part of spiritual rituals, and the young child may imitate the adults. In this case, no diagnosis of pica is warranted. No data have been published about culture-related diagnostic issues that pertain to the other types of atypical eating behaviors.

Gender-Related Diagnostic Issues

Pica may occur in both boys and girls. No specific data regarding gender differences across the other atypical eating behaviors are known.

Differential Diagnosis

Hoarding: Food hoarding requires ruling out hunger.

Pica: If the pica is not severe—and criteria are met for Autism Spectrum Disorder, an intellectual disability, early childhood onset schizophrenia, or Kleine–Levin syndrome—the diagnosis of pica will not be warranted.

Rumination: Common medical conditions in infancy—such as gastro-esophageal reflux, vomiting, pyloric stenosis, hiatal hernia, and Sandifer syndrome—need to be ruled out (by physical examination, x-rays, and laboratory tests).

Comorbidity

Hoarding: Hoarding diagnosis may be comorbid with Obsessive Compulsive Disorder.

Pica: Autism Spectrum Disorder, an intellectual disability, and Kleine–Levin syndrome are comorbid diagnoses commonly seen with pica. Pica also may be associated with Trichotillomania (hair pulling and swallowing) and Skin Picking Disorder.

Rumination: Neurodevelopmental disorder and intellectual disability are often comorbid diagnoses.

Links to DSM–5 and ICD–10

Hoarding: **DSM–5:** Unspecified Feeding or Eating Disorder
ICD–10: Feeding Disorder of Infancy and Early Childhood (F98.2)

Pica: **DSM–5:** Pica
ICD–10: Pica of Infancy and Childhood (F98.3)

Rumination: **DSM–5:** Rumination Disorder
ICD–10: Rumination Disorder of Infancy (F98.21)

Crying Disorder of Infancy/Early Childhood

Introduction

Crying is an innate vocal signal of distress—physical or emotional—essential for survival, especially in the preverbal period of life. Therefore, in isolation, crying is not a disorder. It does become a symptom and a reason for referral to clinicians when the infant/young child goes on crying after his or her needs for food, physical closeness, safety, and regulation have been met by caregivers.

Pediatric handbooks refer to excessive crying as "infant colic" and describe it as a benign, self-limited phenomenon. In spite of the fact that clinicians do encounter severe cases of excessive persistent crying with significant functional impairment, research is sparse, and case descriptions are practically nonexistent.

60.8 Excessive Crying Disorder

Diagnostic Algorithm

All of the following criteria must be met.

A. The infant/young child cries at least 3 hours a day, 3 or more days a week, for at least 3 weeks ("rule of threes").

B. Crying is not better explained by a medical condition (e.g., lactose intolerance, gastroesophageal reflux).

C. Symptoms of the disorder, or caregiver accommodations in response to the symptoms, significantly affect the infant's/young child's and family's functioning in one or more of the following ways:

1. Cause distress to the infant/young child;

2. Interfere with the infant's/young child's relationships;

3. Limit the infant's/young child's participation in developmentally expected activities or routines;

4. Limit the family's participation in everyday activities or routines; or

5. Limit the infant's/young child's ability to learn and develop new skills or interfere with developmental progress.

Diagnostic Features

The infant's/young child's unexplained hyperphonic/dysphonic crying, inconsolability, and fussiness for long bouts of time are the main features of this disorder. The disorder typically starts in the first months of life and goes beyond the commonly known infant colic of the first 3 months of life. The bouts of crying are often accompanied by knee flexion, hypertonic extremities, overinflated abdomen, and reddened face.

Associated Features Supporting Diagnosis

Typically, parents report the infant's/young child's preference for upright position and refusal of horizontal positions as well as the infant's/young child's difficulty to calm down even when held in their arms. Late afternoon and evenings are worse than mornings. This situation inevitably creates a significant overload on the parents; how they react is a function of their coping mechanisms and individual characteristics.

Developmental Features

This disorder is inherently linked to the preverbal period of development and, more specifically, to the first year of life.

Prevalence

Excessive crying during the first 3 months of life has been reported to range between 16% and 29%, depending on the definitions and methods of assessment.

Course

Excessive crying that persists beyond 3 months has its own dynamics: It usually becomes accompanied with parent–infant/young child interactional failure, commencing a vicious cycle. Nights may also become problematic. Over the long run, follow-up studies of young children up to 3 years old have shown typical motor, cognitive, and social development. On the behavioral level, the data are controversial, and it seems that unfavorable prognosis is most evident in studies conducted in clinical samples.

Risk and Prognostic Features

Poor parental self-esteem, lack of intuitive parenting skills, and parental psychopathology are risk factors for the maintenance or the aggravation of excessive crying during and beyond the first 3 months of life. They are also risk factors for the development of seriously disturbed parent–infant/young child relationships, up to the point of physical abuse (e.g., "shaken baby syndrome").

Culture-Related Diagnostic Issues

To the best of our knowledge, there are no data about excessive crying in non-Western countries or in different ethnic groups. One may assume, though, that crying has different meanings across cultures, thus provoking different patterns of response among parents.

Gender-Related Diagnostic Issues

Large studies have not confirmed the common clinical impression that male infants are more prone to excessive crying.

Differential Diagnosis

Difficult temperament, Sensory Processing Disorder, depression, and Deprivation Disorder must be ruled out.

Comorbidity

Sensory Over-Responsivity Disorder, various sleep disorders, and Relationship Specific Disorder of Infancy/Early Childhood may be comorbid with Excessive Crying Disorder.

Links to DSM–5 and ICD–10

DSM–5: N/A
ICD–10: Nonspecific Symptoms Peculiar to Infancy (Excessive Crying in Infants) (R68.11)

60.9 Other Sleep, Eating, and Excessive Crying Disorder of Infancy/Early Childhood

Diagnostic Algorithm

All of the following criteria must be met.

A. The infant/young child has one or more symptoms of a sleep, eating, or crying disorder but does not meet full criteria for the diagnosis.

B. Symptoms of the disorder, or caregiver accommodations in response to the symptoms, significantly affect the infant's/young child's and family's functioning in one or more of the following ways:

  1. Cause distress to the infant/young child;

  2. Interfere with the infant's/young child's relationships;

  3. Limit the infant's/young child's participation in developmentally expected activities or routines;

  4. Limit the family's participation in everyday activities or routines; or

  5. Limit the infant's/young child's ability to learn and develop new skills or interfere with developmental progress.

Specify:

1. The disorder that best explains the infant's/young child's symptoms

2. Why the infant/young child does not meet full criteria

Links to DSM–5 and ICD–10

Feeding-Related: **DSM–5:** Other Specified Feeding or Eating Disorder
ICD–10: Other Eating Disorders (F50.8)

Sleep-Related: **DSM–5:** Other Specified Sleep-Wake Disorder
ICD–10: Other Non-Organic Sleep Disorders (F51.8))

Crying-Related: **DSM–5:** N/A
ICD–10: Nonspecific Symptoms Peculiar to Infancy
(Excessive Crying in Infants) (R68.11)

Most disorders in this manual are defined descriptively without regard to etiology; however, the disorders in this section are an exception to that general rule because each disorder includes an etiology that is specified in the diagnostic criteria. Essentially, this section defines symptomatic behavior that derives from (a) the presence of stressors and traumas (in the case of Posttraumatic Stress Disorder and Adjustment Disorder), (b) the absence of necessary stimulation (in the case of Reactive Attachment Disorder and Disinhibited Social Engagement Disorder), and (c) the loss of a primary caregiving relationship (in the case of Complicated Grief Disorder of Infancy/Early Childhood).

Many of the symptomatic behaviors displayed in these disorders are nonspecific (e.g., aggression, irritability, reduced positive expression of emotions); therefore, linking the behaviors to an etiology of loss, stress, trauma, or deprivation is essential for proper diagnosis. Consequently, it is important to assess for losses, stressors, and traumas in relation to the clinical symptom picture. However, there is abundant evidence that not all infants/young children exposed to stressors, traumas, or deprivation will develop these or any other symptoms. Therefore, in infants/young children who have had such exposures, it is also important to inquire about the specific symptoms that are causing difficulties rather than assuming that exposure equals disorder.

The specific symptoms displayed may vary with the age of the infant/young child, and there are challenges in identifying many of these disorders in the first year of life. For example, Reactive Attachment Disorder and Disinhibited Social Engagement Disorder cannot be diagnosed until after the infant/young child is old enough to have formed a focused attachment. Complicated Grief Disorder of Infancy/Early Childhood also would not be anticipated prior to formation of a focused attachment. Posttraumatic Stress Disorder is challenging to identify in the first year of life because of limited capacities of infants to convey symptoms of re-experiencing. Adjustment Disorder may occur at any age, and it can be considered for symptomatic reactions in the first year of life that are not covered by other disorders in this section, with the understanding that in Adjustment Disorder, symptom expression is limited to 3 months. If symptoms and impairment resulting from trauma, stress, deprivation, or loss extend beyond 3 months and do not meet criteria for another major disorder in this section, Other Trauma, Stress, and Deprivation Disorder of Infancy/Early Childhood is appropriate.

70.1 Posttraumatic Stress Disorder

Introduction

Although exposure to trauma may lead to a number of different disorders, Posttraumatic Stress Disorder (PTSD) describes a specific constellation of symptomatic responses to traumatic exposure. In infants/young children, PTSD always requires exposure to a frightening/terrifying event or a series of events, such as exposure to physical or sexual abuse, intimate partner or community violence, natural disasters, armed conflict, motor vehicle accidents, painful and frightening medical procedures, or similar events. The infant/young child may experience the event directly, witness it as it occurred to others, or learn that the event occurred to a significant person in the infant's/young child's life. The defining feature is a characteristic set of signs that appear following the exposure. In some infants/young children, a fear-based, re-experiencing clinical picture predominates, especially in response to a single discrete traumatic event. A picture of withdrawal and reduced responsiveness predominates in other infants/young children, especially those exposed to chronically traumatic circumstances.

Diagnostic Algorithm

In addition to trauma exposure as specified in criterion A, the following symptoms must be present: at least one symptom from cluster B, at least one symptom from either cluster C or cluster D, and at least two symptoms from cluster E. In addition, the conditions described in criterion F must be present.

A. The infant/young child was exposed to significant threat of or actual serious injury, accident, illness, medical trauma, significant loss, disaster, violence (e.g., partner violence, community violence, war or terrorism), or physical/sexual abuse in one or more of the following ways:

1. Directly experiencing the traumatic event.

2. Hearing or seeing, in person, the event as it occurred to others.

3. Learning that the traumatic event occurred to a significant person in the infant's/young child's life.

B. The infant/young child shows evidence of re-experiencing the traumatic event(s) by demonstrating at least one of the following:

1. Play or behavior that reenacts some aspect of the trauma(s).

2. Preoccupation with the traumatic event(s) conveyed by repeated statements or questions about some aspect of the event(s). Distress is not necessarily apparent.

3. Repeated nightmares, the content of which may or may not be linked to the traumatic event(s), which increase in frequency after the traumatic event(s).

4. Significant distress at reminders of the traumatic event(s).

5. Marked physiological reactions (e.g., sweating, agitated breathing, changes in color) at reminders of the traumatic event(s).

6. Dissociative episodes, beginning after the traumatic event(s), in which the infant/young child freezes, stills, or stares and is unresponsive to environmental stimuli for seconds to minutes in response to reminders of the traumatic event(s).

C. The infant/young child persistently attempts to avoid trauma-related stimuli through efforts to avoid people, places, activities, conversations, or interpersonal situations that are reminders of the trauma(s).

D. The infant/young child experiences a dampening of positive emotional responsiveness that appears or intensifies after the trauma(s) and is revealed by at least one of the following:

1. Increased social withdrawal.

2. Reduced expression of positive emotions.

3. Markedly diminished interest or participation in activities such as play and social interactions.

4. Increased fearfulness or sadness.

E. After a traumatic event, an infant/young child may exhibit onset or intensification of signs of increased arousal, as revealed by at least two of the following:

1. Difficulty going to sleep, evidenced by strong bedtime protest, difficulty falling asleep, or repeated night waking unrelated to nightmares.

2. Difficulty concentrating.

3. Hypervigilance.

4. Exaggerated startle response.

5. Increased irritability, outbursts of anger or extreme fussiness, or temper tantrums.

F. Symptoms of the disorder, or caregiver accommodations in response to the symptoms, significantly affect the infant's/young child's and family's functioning in one or more of the following ways:

1. Cause distress to the infant/young child;

2. Interfere with the infant's/young child's relationships;

3. Limit the infant's/young child's participation in developmentally expected activities or routines;

4. Limit the family's participation in everyday activities or routines; or

5. Limit the infant's/young child's ability to learn and develop new skills or interfere with developmental progress.

Age: The diagnosis should be made with caution in infants less than 12 months old.

Duration: The symptoms in clusters B–E must be present for at least 1 month following the exposure(s) in criterion A.

Diagnostic Features

Following exposure to one or more traumas, the symptom clusters that the infant/young child experiences are the same as in older children and adults, but the manifestations of the symptoms are different. The emphasis in infants/young children is on how symptoms are expressed behaviorally rather than through reports of internal experiences. For example, re-experiencing may be more often expressed by play re-enactments or nightmares rather than by intrusive thoughts or a sense of foreshortened future. Avoidance does occur, but it seems to be less common than in older individuals, in part because of infants'/young children's lack of control over their exposure to frightening reminders. In addition, some infants/young children who are traumatized seem to become preoccupied with, rather than avoiding, reminders of the trauma (e.g., a young child attacked by a dog who talks about dogs repeatedly following the attack). Negative thoughts and emotions may be expressed by increased irritability, emotional withdrawal, or seeming detachment.

Associated Features Supporting Diagnosis

Trauma may have many effects on infants/young children other than PTSD. Common effects include new onset of fears and fearfulness or new onset of angry and aggressive behavior. Oppositional behavior is often a feature, as is separation anxiety. Developmental regression or loss of previously acquired skills (e.g., toilet training) may be evident. Some infants/young children with nascent expressive language skills may retain their skills but show selective regression when referencing the traumatic experience.

Developmental Features

PTSD has been described in infants as young as 12 months. Infants younger than 12 months have limited representational capacities, which may be necessary for re-experiencing to occur and to be expressed. Infants in the first year of life may become symptomatic following exposure to a traumatic event, but they are less likely than young children older than 12 months to manifest all the symptoms of PTSD.

Prevalence

PTSD is uncommon in infants/young children in community samples. Rates of PTSD following exposure to trauma vary widely across studies, but overall a minority of infants/young children exposed to serious trauma develop the diagnosis. It is likely that PTSD is under-recognized in infants/young children because infants'/young children's rates of exposures to major stressors and trauma are much higher than the number of infants/young children brought in for assessment and treatment.

Course

The limited available evidence suggests no significant diminution of PTSD symptomatology in infants/young children within the first 2 years following exposure to trauma. The long-term course of PTSD into middle childhood and adolescence is unknown.

Risk and Prognostic Features

Few studies have addressed vulnerability factors for PTSD in infants/young children who have been exposed to traumas. One factor that has preliminary support is that infants/young children exposed to trauma are more likely to develop PTSD if their caregivers are threatened by the same trauma. Studies of biological vulnerability, such as genetic polymorphisms, may be useful in demonstrating risk, although these studies have been notoriously challenging to replicate. An anxious diathesis seems to increase risk for PTSD among older traumatized individuals, and this finding may be true for infants/young children as well, although direct evidence is lacking.

Culture-Related Diagnostic Issues

No cultural differences in the specific clinical picture of PTSD have been demonstrated in infants/young children, although help-seeking, risk of onset, and severity may be affected by cultural beliefs. Indeed, a significant barrier to treatment is the widespread belief among many adult caregivers that infants/young children in the first few years of life are not affected by trauma exposure or that they will outgrow their symptoms.

Gender-Related Diagnostic Issues

No gender differences have been identified for this disorder in infants/young children.

Differential Diagnosis

The clinical picture of PTSD includes both specific and nonspecific symptoms. Specific symptoms are sudden onset of distressing symptoms following exposure to trauma and, especially, re-experiencing the traumatic event in various ways. Nonspecific symptoms are negative effects, including irritability, fearfulness, and emotional withdrawal. Onset or intensification of symptoms following exposure to a trauma is necessary to meet criteria for a diagnosis of PTSD. Adjustment Disorder is appropriate if the infant/young child has experienced a trauma and has symptoms for less than 3 months but does not meet criteria for PTSD. For infants/young children who are traumatized and do not meet criteria for PTSD and whose symptoms extend beyond 3 months, a diagnosis of Other Trauma, Stress, and Deprivation Disorder of Infancy/Early Childhood is appropriate.

Comorbidity

The comorbidity pattern for PTSD in infants/young children is somewhat different than for older children, adolescents, and adults. Oppositional behavior and separation anxiety are especially common, especially in clinical samples.

For infants/young children who experience maltreatment, cognitive, language, and motor delays are common.

Links to DSM–5 and ICD–10

DSM–5: Posttraumatic Stress Disorder for Children 6 Years and Younger
ICD–10: Post-Traumatic Stress Disorder (F43.10)

70.2 Adjustment Disorder

Introduction

Adjustment Disorder describes a condition in which an infant/young child develops symptoms in response to one or more stressors. The stressors may be acute, chronic, or enduring circumstances, and the symptomatic picture is less than 3 months. The diagnosis of Adjustment Disorder should be considered for any situational disturbance that is not better explained by another Axis I disorder, that is not merely an exacerbation of a preexisting disorder, and that does not represent developmentally appropriate reactions to changes in the environment.

Diagnostic Algorithm

All of the following criteria must be met.

A. One or more significant new environmental stressors have occurred.

B. Within 2 weeks of exposure to the stressor, the infant/young child exhibits a disturbance of emotions (e.g., irritability, sadness, soberness, or anxiety) or behaviors (e.g., oppositionality, resistance to going to sleep, frequent tantrums, or developmental regression).

C. The emotional or behavioral disturbances in criterion B represent a clear change in emotions or behavior and seem plausibly related to the stressor.

D. Symptomatic responses to a stressor are not:

   1. Better explained by another Axis I disorder.

   2. Merely an exacerbation of a preexisting disorder.

   3. Developmentally appropriate reactions to changes in the environment.

E. Symptoms of the disorder, or caregiver accommodations in response to the symptoms, significantly affect the infant's/young child's and family's functioning in one or more of the following ways:

   1. Cause distress to the infant/young child;

   2. Interfere with the infant's/young child's relationships;

   3. Limit the infant's/young child's participation in developmentally expected activities or routines;

4. Limit the family's participation in everyday activities or routines; or

5. Limit the infant's/young child's ability to learn and develop new skills or interfere with developmental progress.

Age: There are no age specifications.

Duration: The symptoms must be present for at least 2 weeks and for less than 3 months if the stressor is no longer present.

Diagnostic Features

The essential features of Adjustment Disorder require an identifiable environmental stressor and a symptomatic response to that stressor or circumstance that does not meet criteria for another Axis I disorder. If the infant's/young child's symptomatic behavior is better accounted for by another disorder, Adjustment Disorder is ruled out. The clinical presentation varies widely, ranging from disturbances in emotion regulation (e.g., frequent crying), to disturbances of physiological regulation (e.g., sleep refusal), to behavioral manifestations (e.g., hyperactivity), or to some combination. The requirement that the symptoms manifest for at least 2 weeks is an effort to distinguish the disorder from transient developmental perturbations. The disorder limits the infant's/young child's ability to engage in developmentally appropriate activities and to engage fully in interaction with adults and peers.

Associated Features Supporting Diagnosis

There are no known associated features for Adjustment Disorder in infants/young children because the symptoms are variable and nonspecific.

Developmental Features

Infants have a narrower range of behavioral repertoire than young children, and their symptomatic expressions are likely to be more limited. Infants may exhibit symptoms such as sleep disturbances, eating problems, social withdrawal, or excessive crying—all of which would have to be subthreshold for the Axis I disorders that involve those behaviors. Young children may exhibit any of these symptoms, plus others such as hyperactivity, oppositional behavior, or aggression.

Prevalence

The prevalence of Adjustment Disorder in infants/young children is not known but is believed to be common.

Course

Adjustment Disorder is often thought to be limited, although there are no defined boundaries in infants/young children. The paucity of longitudinal data about the natural history of Adjustment Disorder makes it unclear how to describe the course.

Risk and Prognostic Features

Individual risk factors likely vary depending on the type of environmental stressor or circumstance. Although significant stressors occur across environmental contexts, infants/young children living in higher risk environments are at greater risk for Adjustment Disorder.

Culture-Related Diagnostic Issues

Cultural differences in psychiatric symptomatology and in the meaning ascribed to behaviors and expressions of emotions are well documented in older individuals but are not well studied in infants/young children. Clinicians should evaluate the clinical presentation in the context of the infant's/young child's culture for reference to adaptive versus maladaptive behavioral responses and to determine whether the response is excessive.

Gender-Related Diagnostic Issues

There are no known differences between boys and girls with regard to Adjustment Disorder in infancy/early childhood.

Differential Diagnosis

Adjustment Disorder defines symptomatic behaviors in the infant/young child that are not better accounted for by another Axis I disorder. Stressors are ubiquitous, and the presence of symptomatic behavior in the context of an acute or chronic stressor or more enduring environmental circumstance does not necessarily indicate presence of Adjustment Disorder. If the stressor does not account for the symptomatic response, as when stressors or traumas exacerbate preexisting disorders, Adjustment Disorder is not diagnosed. Furthermore, if the infant/young child is exposed to trauma and develops Posttraumatic Stress Disorder (PTSD), Adjustment Disorder is ruled out. Similarly, if the infant/young child experiences a significant interpersonal loss and manifests Complicated Grief Disorder of Infancy/Early Childhood, Adjustment Disorder is ruled out. Adjustment Disorder may be appropriate for subthreshold manifestations of these disorders, however, such as an infant/young child who is traumatized, symptomatic, and impaired but who does not meet all criteria for PTSD.

Comorbidity

Adjustment Disorder may accompany any other disorder or medical condition, but it should include symptoms not accounted for by the comorbid disorder. Co-occurrence of Adjustment Disorder and another Axis I disorder must be distinguished from an exacerbation of a preexisting condition. For example, a young child with Attention Deficit Hyperactivity Disorder may become fearful and irritable after being in an automobile accident. If the young child does not meet criteria for PTSD, Adjustment Disorder should be considered.

Links to DSM–5 and ICD–10

DSM–5: Adjustment Disorder
ICD–10: Adjustment Disorder Unspecified (F43.20)

70.3 Complicated Grief Disorder of Infancy/ Early Childhood

Introduction

The death or permanent loss of an attachment figure represents a severe emotional stressor for an infant/young child. Infants/young children have not yet developed an understanding of the permanence of death and the involuntary nature of most deaths, and their effort to give meaning to the absence of the loved one reflects the cognitive capacities and limitations of their developmental stage. In infants, emotional distress and somatic manifestations—such as disturbances in feeding, sleeping, and digestive processes—predominate. Young children construct explanations for the death or permanent loss that may involve self-attributions, such as causing the attachment figure's death because of their anger or behavior. The infant's/young child's difficulty in creating a reality-based understanding of the death/permanent loss may result in pathogenic beliefs, such as being unlovable or negative emotions being dangerous, that have a deleterious effect on the infant's/young child's healthy developmental trajectory. The circumstances of the death/permanent loss and the availability of consistent and supportive alternative attachment figures are important factors in determining the course of the infant's/young child's mourning process. Most infants/young children are able to tolerate their intense distress, create a developmentally appropriate explanation of the death, and redirect their attachment to substitute adults when they are supported in these processes by their remaining primary caregivers. The category of Complicated Grief Disorder of Infancy/Early Childhood is designed for those infants/ young children who show a significant and pervasive impairment of function following a death/permanent loss that lasts for at least 30 days and interferes with normative developmental activities.

Diagnostic Algorithm

All of the following criteria must be met.

A. Following the death or permanent loss of an attachment figure, the infant/ young child exhibits at least two of the following symptoms:

1. The infant/young child persistently cries, calls, or searches for the lost person.

2. When encountering reminders of the loss, the infant/young child shows any of the following:

    a. Detachment, including seeming indifferent toward reminders of the caregiver, such as a photograph or mention of the caregiver's name.

    b. Selective "forgetting," including apparent lack of recognition of photographs or other reminders of the lost person.

    c. Extreme sensitivity to any reminder of the lost person, including acute distress when a possession that belonged to the person is touched by another or is taken away.

    d. A strong emotional reaction to any theme connected with separation and loss—for example, refusal to play hide-and-seek, bursting into tears when a household object is moved from its customary place, intense separation distress, or persistent preoccupation with the whereabouts of others.

  3. Persistent preoccupation with the possible death of self or others, such as any of the following:

    a. Repeated questions about dying ("Will I die?" "Will you die?").

    b. Statements about wishing to die ("I want to die, too") or play enactment of death themes.

    c. Repeatedly telling strangers about the loss of caregiver.

B. The infant's/young child's reaction to the loss includes three or more of the following:

  1. Fatigue or loss of energy.

  2. Depressed affect or sad facial expression.

  3. Lack of interest in age-appropriate activities.

  4. Self-harming or self-endangering behaviors.

  5. Statements that denote guilt or self-blame about the loss (e.g., "I am bad"; "I killed him [or her]").

  6. Significant sleep changes.

  7. Significant eating/feeding changes.

  8. Loss of developmental milestones.

C. Symptoms of the disorder, or caregiver accommodations in response to the symptoms, significantly affect the infant's/young child's and family's functioning in one or more of the following ways:

  1. Cause distress to the infant/young child;

  2. Interfere with the infant's/young child's relationships;

  3. Limit the infant's/young child's participation in developmentally expected activities or routines;

  4. Limit the family's participation in everyday activities or routines; or

  5. Limit the infant's/young child's ability to learn and develop new skills or interfere with developmental progress.

Age: No minimum age is specified, but the diagnosis should be made with caution in infants less than 9 months old (the developmental age at which preferred attachment should be clearly established).

Duration: The symptoms must be present more days than not for at least 30 days.

Specify:

1. Whether the infant/young child was present during the events leading to the death
2. Whether the infant/young child was exposed to information about the circumstances of the death

Diagnostic Features

Complicated Grief Disorder of Infancy/Early Childhood is diagnosed only if the symptoms listed previously are present more days than not for at least 30 days. This pattern of pervasiveness and persistence differentiates this diagnosis from infants'/young children's normative grieving patterns, which may be characterized by intense distress, preoccupation with the whereabouts of the person who died, or other manifestations of grieving that are usually circumscribed in duration and do not interfere significantly with the infant's/young child's developmental course and everyday functioning. In preverbal infants/young children, symptoms are expressed somatically, behaviorally, or through emotional responses. The nature and severity of grief must exceed expected norms for the infant's/young child's developmental stage and cultural group and be impairing for the infant/young child.

Associated Features Supporting Diagnosis

The death/permanent loss of an attachment figure may have effects on infants/young children other than complex grief. The infant/young child may become fearful of becoming attached to other adults for fear that they will also die; may avoid activities because of fear that they may result in injury or death; and may show reduced interest in exploration, learning, and problem solving. Role reversal may occur, with young children becoming precociously solicitous about the well-being of caregivers because of fear for their safety. Separation anxiety is usually exacerbated following loss or permanent separation from an attachment figure.

Developmental Features

There are no systematic studies of the course of grief in infants/young children less than 3 years old, and there are very few studies involving preschool-age young children. Infants in the first year of life may be intensely distressed by permanent separation or loss of an attachment figure, which they are likely to express through crying, lack of soothability, sleep disruptions, and listlessness. Young children may develop self-attributions about causing the death, preoccupation with death and dying, worry about having caused the death, negative thoughts such as wishing to die to join the attachment figure, and anger or ambivalent attachment involving substitute caregivers.

Prevalence

No data are available about the prevalence of Complicated Grief Disorder of Infancy/Early Childhood.

Course

The long-term course of Complicated Grief Disorder of Infancy/Early Childhood is not known.

Risk and Prognostic Features

Clinical experience suggests that infants/young children who have surviving alternative attachment figures are less likely to develop a disorder than those who lose their only attachment figure. There is some indication that infants/young children who lost an attachment figure in infancy/early childhood may be more prone to react with depression in later life following the loss of a loved person.

Culture-Related Diagnostic Issues

There are no studies addressing cultural differences in the manifestation of Complicated Grief Disorder of Infancy/Early Childhood in infants/young children. A significant obstacle to these studies is the pervasive belief across different cultural groups that infants/young children will forget the person who died/lost if the person is not mentioned and if reminders of the person are removed from the infant's/young child's everyday environment.

Gender-Related Diagnostic Issues

No gender differences have been identified for this disorder in infants/young children.

Differential Diagnosis

The clinical picture of Complicated Grief Disorder of Infancy/Early Childhood includes specific and nonspecific symptoms. Specific symptoms are sudden onset of distressing symptoms following the loss, as described in the criteria for the disorder. Nonspecific symptoms are negative affect, including pervasive sadness, irritability, fearfulness, and emotional withdrawal. Onset or intensification of symptoms following the death or permanent loss is necessary to meet criteria for a diagnosis of Complicated Grief Disorder of Infancy/Early Childhood. A diagnosis of Adjustment Disorder involves primarily a nonspecific emotional or behavioral response to a traumatic or stressful event without symptoms involving preoccupation with loss or death.

Comorbidity

There are no studies documenting comorbidity of Complicated Grief Disorder of Infancy/Early Childhood. Features of Generalized Anxiety Disorder and Depressive Disorder of Early Childhood have been observed clinically.

Links to DSM–5 and ICD–10

DSM–5: Other Specified Trauma- and Stressor-Related Disorder
(Persistent Complex Bereavement Disorder)
ICD–10: Other Reactions to Severe Stress (F43.8)

70.4 Reactive Attachment Disorder

Introduction

Reactive Attachment Disorder (RAD) describes a condition in an infant/young child who lacks an attachment figure, despite being developmentally capable of forming an attachment. Infants/young children are born with a strong propensity to form attachments to caregiving adults, and they do except in unusual circumstances in which they lack sufficient social interaction with caregivers. Manifestations of the disorder include both lack of expected attachment behaviors and aberrant social and emotional responsiveness. This disorder is diagnosed by detailed history and observation of an infant's/young child's behaviors during a clinical assessment. There are no specific tests or procedures indicated to confirm or support the diagnosis.

Diagnostic Algorithm

All of the following criteria must be met.

A. Lack of attachment to any caregiving adult that manifests as:

1. A pattern of emotionally withdrawn, inhibited behavior with adult caregivers that is characterized by at least two of the following:

   a. Absent or significantly reduced interest in engaging socially with others.

   b. Absent or significantly reduced developmentally appropriate comfort seeking when distressed.

   c. Absent or significantly reduced responses to comfort when offered.

   d. Absent or significantly reduced social reciprocity with adult caregivers.

2. A pattern of emotion regulation difficulties characterized by reduced or absent positive affect and episodes of excessive or unexplained fearfulness or irritability/anger with caregivers.

B. The lack of an attachment figure results from the infant/young child experiencing insufficient care (social and emotional neglect) or repeated changes in caregivers that limit the infant's/young child's ability to form attachments and resulting in the anomalous behaviors in criterion A1.

C. The criteria are not met for Autism Spectrum Disorder (ASD) or Early Atypical Autism Spectrum Disorder (EAASD).

D. Symptoms of the disorder, or caregiver accommodations in response to the symptoms, significantly affect the infant's/young child's and family's functioning in one or more of the following ways:

1. Cause distress to the infant/young child;

2. Interfere with the infant's/young child's relationships;

3. Limit the infant's/young child's participation in developmentally expected activities or routines;

4. Limit the family's participation in everyday activities or routines; or

5. Limit the infant's/young child's ability to learn and develop new skills or interfere with developmental progress.

Age: The disorder may not be diagnosed in infants with a developmental age of less than 9 months.

Duration: There is no minimum duration required.

Diagnostic Features

The essence of this disorder is the absence of an attachment to any caregiving adult in infants/young children who have experienced serious social neglect. The infant/young child must be old enough to have formed a selective attachment— that is, have a cognitive age of at least 9 months. The absence of attachment behaviors, such as seeking comfort, support, nurturance, and protection, also are evident by the lack of stranger wariness (because the infant/young child may be wary of all adults) and the lack of separation protest. In addition, the infant/young child demonstrates reduced or absent social reciprocity during interactions and emotion regulation disturbances that include reduced positive emotions and unexplained episodes of fear, irritability, or sadness. There is an overall quality of withdrawal and an inhibition of expected attachment behaviors in the infant/young child that are evident cross-contextually.

Associated Features Supporting Diagnosis

The disorder seriously limits the infant's/young child's ability to seek and obtain comfort for distress and to enjoy social interaction with adults and peers. Because infants/young children with RAD have experienced social neglect, they also often manifest other problems, such as cognitive, language, and motor delays; stereotypies; and growth delays, including height, weight, and head circumference.

Developmental Features

After an infant has reached a cognitive age of 9 months old, it is anticipated that the infant will exhibit preferences for a relatively small number of caregiving adults. Proximity-seeking behaviors in older infants/young children may include crawling or ambulating to a caregiver, clinging on to a caregiver, smiling or crying to elicit physical closeness, leaning in for contact, and other similar behaviors. As young children get older, many of these behaviors persist, but verbal exchanges are also used to elicit closeness and express the need for comfort. Bearing in mind differences in how attachment behaviors are expressed from 9 months to 5 years old, the essential manifestations of RAD are similar throughout this period.

Prevalence

The disorder is rare. In community samples, it is usually not reported. Even in high-risk samples of infants/young children who have experienced social neglect or who have been raised in impersonal institutions, most infants/young children do not manifest RAD.

Course

The limited data that are available suggest that if conditions of deprivation persist, infants/young children continue to manifest signs of RAD. The disorder is quite responsive to adequate caregiving environments, and on the basis of studies of infants/young children placed in foster care or adopted from depriving institutions, signs of the disorder diminish within weeks of removal from the neglectful environment and placement in an adequate environment.

Risk and Prognostic Features

Although a minority of infants/young children exposed to severe social neglect will develop RAD, little is known about why some do and others do not manifest RAD. It appears to require neglect in the earliest years, perhaps even before the first attachment forms, but studies are limited on this point. Within the first 3 years of life, it does not seem to matter at what point the infant/young child is removed from the neglectful environment because signs of the disorder diminish or disappear quickly regardless of the infant's/young child's age. What is less clear is whether, after the disorder is no longer apparent, the infant/young child is at risk for subsequent problems in relatedness and attachment. Given the centrality of attachment in early social and emotional development, RAD should be considered a developmental emergency, and efforts to place infants/young children who show signs of this disorder into adequate (or better) caregiving environments should be an urgent priority.

Culture-Related Diagnostic Issues

Data are too limited at this point to know about cultural differences in the prevalence, course, or clinical presentation of RAD.

Gender-Related Diagnostic Issues

There are no known differences in RAD related to gender.

Differential Diagnosis

ASD and EAASD both involve infants/young children with aberrant social behaviors, dampened expression of positive emotions, cognitive and language delays, and impairments in social reciprocity. In addition, both disorders may be associated with developmental delays and stereotypic motor behaviors. These disorders must be ruled out before a diagnosis of RAD can be made.

Despite broad similarities, there are a number of ways in which RAD differs from these neurodevelopmental disorders. First, ASD and EAASD should not ordinarily involve a history of neglect. Second, restricted and repetitive behaviors; excessive adherence to rituals and routines; restricted, fixated interests; and unusual sensory reactions should not be present in RAD. Third, although RAD may occur with developmental delays, both ASD and EAASD involve selective delays in social communicative behaviors—such as intentional communication—and in pretend play that are more impaired than their overall intellectual functioning. Infants/young children with RAD, however, should have social communicative skills that are comparable with their overall level of cognitive functioning. Finally, considerable research has demonstrated that young children with ASD often demonstrate attachment behaviors, whereas infants/young children with RAD do so only rarely or inconsistently.

Infants/young children with intellectual disabilities may share an even profile of delayed cognitive and motor skills and milestones with infants/young children with RAD. Nevertheless, there is no reason to expect abnormal social and emotional behaviors and responsiveness in infants/young children with intellectual disabilities. They should form attachments to caregiving adults when they reach a cognitive age of 7–9 months. Infants/young children with RAD, however, show selective impairments of social and emotional responsiveness and an absence of preferred attachments despite having attained a cognitive age of at least 9 months old.

Depression and RAD in young children are both associated with reductions in positive affect, and with anhedonia. However, there is no reason to expect that depression alone should inhibit attachment behaviors. Young children who have a diagnosis of a depressive disorder should seek and respond to comforting efforts by caregivers, although the available data are limited.

Comorbidity

RAD frequently co-occurs with cognitive and language delays (both expressive and receptive delays). Motor delays sometimes occur, as do motor abnormalities, such as stereotypies or problems with balance and coordination. Height, weight, and head circumference are sometimes reduced, and malnutrition may occur if physical neglect is also present. Symptoms of depression frequently are evident.

Links to DSM–5 and ICD–10

DSM–5: Reactive Attachment Disorder
ICD–10: Reactive Attachment Disorder (F94.1)

70.5 Disinhibited Social Engagement Disorder

Introduction

Disinhibited Social Engagement Disorder (DSED) defines a pattern of socially aberrant behavior with unfamiliar adults in an infant/young child who has experienced serious social neglect. It is characterized by reduced or absent reticence about approaching and engaging with unfamiliar adults. In typically developing infants/young children, stranger wariness ordinarily appears in the latter part of the first year of life and continues to be evident in varying degrees through the second and third years, with gradual waning in the preschool years. In DSED, there is no or almost no stranger wariness—in fact, there is an active seeking of contact and interaction with unfamiliar adults. Although historically considered an attachment disorder, DSED may occur in infants/young children who lack attachments to anyone or in infants/young children who have established attachments. This disorder is diagnosed by detailed history and observation of an infant's/young child's behaviors during a clinical assessment. There are no specific tests or procedures indicated to confirm or support the diagnosis.

Diagnostic Algorithm

All of the following criteria must be met.

A. Recurrent tendency to approach and interact with unfamiliar adults without displaying expected reticence as manifest by at least two of the following:

1. Repeated willingness to depart with unfamiliar adult caregivers without hesitation.

2. Repeated tendency to engage in physically (e.g., touching, hugging) or verbally (e.g., asking overly familiar questions) intrusive interactions that are age inappropriate with unfamiliar adults.

3. Repeated tendency to fail to track an adult caregiver's whereabouts in unfamiliar settings by monitoring, checking back, or staying close.

B. Social disinhibition with adults that is distinct from behavioral impulsivity (i.e., acting without thinking) and that violates culturally accepted developmental norms.

C. The infant/young child has experienced insufficient care (social and emotional neglect) or repeated changes in caregivers that limit the infant's/young child's ability to form attachments. The insufficient care is believed to lead to the anomalous behaviors described in criterion A.

D. Symptoms of the disorder, or caregiver accommodations in response to the symptoms, significantly affect the infant's/young child's and family's functioning in one or more of the following ways:

1. Cause distress to the infant/young child;

2. Interfere with the infant's/young child's relationships;

3. Limit the infant's/young child's participation in developmentally expected activities or routines;

4. Limit the family's participation in everyday activities or routines; or

5. Limit the infant's/young child's ability to learn and develop new skills or interfere with developmental progress.

Age: The disorder may not be diagnosed in infants with a developmental age of less than 9 months and should be diagnosed with caution before 12 months old.

Duration: There is no minimum duration required.

Specify:

1. Whether the infant/young child lacks a fully formed attachment

Diagnostic Features

The essence of this disorder is infants/young children who lack reticence about actively approaching and engaging socially with unfamiliar adults following serious social neglect in the caregiving environment. The infant/young child must be old enough to have developed stranger wariness—that is, have a cognitive age of at least 9 months. The social engagement exhibited by infants/young children with this disorder has been described as "overfriendly," but it is often experienced as intrusive and unwanted. The infant/young child exhibits a pattern of violating social boundaries through excessive physical touch and verbally intrusive questions.

Associated Features Supporting Diagnosis

The disorder may seriously limit the infant's/young child's quality of relationships with important others. Caregivers may describe the infant/young child as emotionally superficial or as attention seeking. There is a possibility of self-endangerment from not remaining physically close to attachment figures in unfamiliar settings or in willingly departing with unknown adults. Because infants/young children with DSED have experienced social neglect, they also often manifest other problems, such as cognitive, language, and motor delays; stereotypies; and growth delays, including height, weight, and head circumference.

Developmental Features

After an infant has reached a cognitive age of 9 months, it is anticipated that the infant will exhibit preferences for a relatively small number of caregiving adults. One behavior that heralds the onset of focused attachment is stranger wariness. Following a period of high interest in social interaction with anyone that is usually evident from about 2–7 months, infants begin to react with distress or at least hesitation about overtures from unfamiliar adults at around 7–9 months. The disorder will be most apparent when young children are able to freely approach and depart with unfamiliar adults, so the diagnosis should be made with caution before 12 months old.

Prevalence

The disorder is rare. In community samples, it is usually not reported. Even in high-risk samples of infants/young children who have experienced social neglect or who have been raised in impersonal institutions, most infants/young children do not manifest DSED.

Course

The limited data that are available suggest that if conditions of deprivation persist, infants/young children continue to manifest signs of DSED. The disorder is not always responsive to adequate caregiving environments. In fact, in infants/young children adopted out of conditions of social and emotional deprivation, indiscriminate behavior is one of the most persistent abnormalities reported. There is suggestive evidence that the sooner an infant/young child is placed in an adequate environment, the more likely that signs of the disorder diminish. Other reasons for persistence or desistance are less clear.

Risk and Prognostic Features

Although a minority of infants/young children exposed to severe social neglect will develop DSED, little is known about why some do and others do not develop the disorder. It appears to require neglect in the earliest years, perhaps even before the first attachment forms, but studies are limited on this point. There is no clear evidence at present that deprivation beginning after the second year of life leads to the disorder, but here again, evidence is limited.

Culture-Related Diagnostic Issues

Data are too limited to know about cultural differences in the prevalence, course, or clinical presentation of DSED.

Gender-Related Diagnostic Issues

There are no known differences in DSED related to gender.

Differential Diagnosis

The first challenge is to determine whether an infant/young child is highly sociable or truly indiscriminate. Some infants/young children are temperamentally disposed to approach and engage with others, and it is important to make this distinction. In more unfamiliar settings, it is expected that infants/young children will be less inclined to wander off or approach unfamiliar adults, so displays of disinhibited social inhibition are more indicative in these instances than when they occur in familiar settings. Also, the more intrusive and unwelcome the social approaches of the infant/young child, the more likely these behaviors are signs of DSED. Nevertheless, it is important to determine that the behaviors are functionally impairing to the infant/young child to confirm the diagnosis.

Young children with Attention Deficit Hyperactivity Disorder (ADHD) demonstrate impulsivity that may extend to social interactions. Careful assessment should include whether the young child's impulsivity includes cognitive (e.g., inhibitory control problems), behavioral (e.g., running into the street without looking), or social (e.g., requesting to sit on the lap of an unfamiliar adult) disinhibition. There is no reason to expect nonsocial impulsivity in young children with DSED, although it may co-occur with ADHD.

Young children with intellectual disabilities also may exhibit some aspects of indiscriminate behavior, perhaps related to having reduced judgment about social boundaries. If DSED is present, the social boundary violations should be out of proportion to the young child's developmental level and other problems with judgment.

Comorbidity

DSED may co-occur with other problems known to result from deprivation, including cognitive and language delays, motor delays, stereotypies, problems with balance and coordination, growth problems, and ADHD. In addition, signs of externalizing behavior problems, including aggression, may co-occur with DSED.

70.6 Other Trauma, Stress, and Deprivation Disorder of Infancy/Early Childhood

Diagnostic Algorithm

All of the following criteria must be met.

A. The infant/young child has one or more symptoms of a trauma, stress, or deprivation disorder but does not meet full criteria for the diagnosis.

B. Symptoms of the disorder, or caregiver accommodations in response to the symptoms, significantly affect the infant's/young child's and family's functioning in one or more of the following ways:

1. Cause distress to the infant/young child;

2. Interfere with the infant's/young child's relationships;

3. Limit the infant's/young child's participation in developmentally expected activities or routines;

4. Limit the family's participation in everyday activities or routines; or

5. Limit the infant's/young child's ability to learn and develop new skills or interfere with developmental progress.

Specify:

1. The disorder that best explains the infant's/young child's symptoms

2. Why the infant/young child does not meet full criteria

Links to DSM–5 and ICD–10

DSM–5: Unspecified Trauma- and Stressor-Related Disorder
ICD–10: Reaction to Severe Stress, Unspecified (F43.9)

Historically, psychiatry and medicine have defined disorders as existing within individuals. Implicit in this tradition is the expectation that the symptomatic behavior will be expressed cross-contextually and in all relationships. Although there may be some variation in the intensity of symptom expression, the disorder is carried by that individual, and therefore, the symptoms are specific to the individual and expressed similarly across contexts and relationships.

Research on relationships between infants/young children and their caregivers, however, has demonstrated that behaviors of infants/young children may differ systematically with different caregivers. Within the first few months of life, infants demonstrate distinctive and somewhat stable patterns of interacting with different caregivers. By the end of the first year, they may demonstrate different patterns of attachment to different caregivers. In addition, research paradigms have identified behaviors in infants as young as 3 months old as "depressed," but it seems that this depressed behavior is relationship specific. There are also numerous case reports of symptomatic behavior in the context of one caregiving relationship that does not generalize to other relationships.

Relationship Specific Disorder of Infancy/Early Childhood describes symptomatic behavior in the infant/young child that is limited to one caregiving relationship. There is no specification for the behaviors that the infant/young child displays but only that these behaviors are evident in one but not in other relationships and that the behaviors impair the infant's/young child's functioning. If the behaviors are evident in more than one context, the disorder cannot be diagnosed. As a newly defined disorder with emerging direct empirical validation, the disorder is conservatively defined; it is considered only if there is affirmative evidence of the symptoms being present in one but not in other relationship contexts. For example, if an infant/young child has sleep refusal at home (with impaired functioning) but does not sleep overnight in other settings, Sleep Onset Disorder rather than Relationship Specific Disorder of Infancy/Early Childhood is appropriate. However, if the infant/young child shows no sleep refusal in his or her grandmother's house, where he or she sleeps several times a week, then the sleep refusal at home would meet criteria for Relationship Specific Disorder of Infancy/Early Childhood.

By focusing on infant/young child symptomatic behavior, this diagnosis does not encompass infants/young children who are only at risk for psychopathology because of the nature of their relationship with a primary caregiver. For example, there is considerable evidence that infants/young children with disorganized attachment behaviors in the strange situation procedure are at risk for concurrent and subsequent psychopathology. Many infants/young children with one or more disorganized attachment relationships also have dysregulated and disordered behavior. Nevertheless, the classification of disorganized attachment—which is identified on the basis of the infant's/young child's behavior in a structured, 20-minute laboratory procedure—is not in and of itself indicative of a disorder. Diagnosing a relationship disorder requires evidence of a persistent emotional or behavioral disturbance and functional impairment. Thus, many infants/young children with a relationship disorder will have disorganized attachments, but some will not; furthermore, some infants/young children with disorganized attachments will have Relationship Specific Disorder of Infancy/ Early Childhood, but others will not.

Because Axis II is designed to characterize the infant's/young child's relationship context, there is a need for clarity about how Axis II and Relationship Specific Disorder of Infancy/Early Childhood interrelate. In particular, Part A: Caregiver–Infant/Young Child Relationship Adaptation under Axis II is most relevant to Relationship Specific Disorder of Infancy/ Early Childhood under Axis I. First, only infants/young children who meet criteria for the Axis I disorder—impairing, symptomatic behavior limited to one relationship context—will receive the diagnosis of Relationship Specific Disorder of Infancy/Early Childhood. In contrast, *all* infants/young children should have their relationship context characterized under Axis II (Parts A and B), with adaptations ranging from exemplary to dangerously disturbed. If the infant/young child is diagnosed with Relationship Specific Disorder of Infancy/ Early Childhood, the rating of the infant's/young child's relationship with the primary caregiver should be Level 3 or Level 4 under Axis II. Second, there is no presumption in Relationship Specific Disorder of Infancy/Early Childhood with regard to the etiology of the symptom picture. Relationship disturbances can arise from problems within the caregiver, the infant/young child, the unique fit between the two, or various combinations of the preceding. In the Axis II section, Table 1 (Dimensions of Caregiving) and Table 2 (Infant's/Young Child's Contributions to the Relationship) can be used to consider more specific contributors, but those considerations are not needed for and not included in the criteria for the Axis I disorder.

80.1 Relationship Specific Disorder of Infancy/ Early Childhood

Introduction

This disorder defines symptomatic behavior in the infant/young child that is limited to one relationship context. For example, a young child who is oppositional only with one preschool teacher, or a young child who exhibits role-inappropriate behavior with the primary caregiver only, would qualify for the diagnosis if the symptomatic behavior is impairing. The disorder derives from the demonstration that although relational disturbances for infants/ young children are not uncommon, they are sometimes expressed through the infant's/young child's behaviors and emotions. Although psychopathology is traditionally defined as existing within an individual rather than between individuals, research and clinical experience indicate that an infant/young child may have very different behaviors in relationships with different caregivers. At one extreme, the infant/young child may exhibit emotional or behavioral symptoms in the context of one particular caregiving relationship but not other relationships. This is the essence of Relationship Specific Disorder of Infancy/Early Childhood, which describes relational disturbances that are manifest in infants'/young children's symptomatic behavior.

Diagnostic Algorithm

All of the following criteria must be met.

A. The infant/young child exhibits a persistent emotional or behavioral disturbance in the context of one particular relationship with a caregiver. Examples include (but are not limited to) the following:

1. Oppositional behavior.

2. Aggression.

3. Fearfulness.

4. Self-endangering behavior.

5. Food refusal.

6. Sleep refusal.

7. Role-inappropriate behavior with caregiver (e.g., over-solicitous or controlling behavior).

B. The symptomatology in criterion A is expressed exclusively in one caregiving relationship.

C. Symptoms of the disorder, or caregiver accommodations in response to the symptoms, significantly affect the infant's/young child's and family's functioning in one or more of the following ways:

1. Cause distress to the infant/young child;

2. Interfere with the infant's/young child's relationships;

3. Limit the infant's/young child's participation in developmentally expected activities or routines;

4. Limit the family's participation in everyday activities or routines; or

5. Limit the infant's/young child's ability to learn and develop new skills or interfere with developmental progress.

Age: There are no age restrictions, but relationship specificity may be difficult to ascertain in the earliest months of life.

Duration: The symptoms must be present for at least 1 month.

Specify:

1. Symptoms that are relationship specific

2. Caregiver(s) with whom symptomatology is manifest

Diagnostic Features

The essential feature of Relationship Specific Disorder of Infancy/Early Childhood is that infants/young children exhibit a pattern of symptomatic behavior in the context of one caregiver relationship but not in others, and the symptomatic behavior is associated with functional impairment. Diagnosing this disorder requires affirmative evidence of relationship specificity. In the case of an infant/young child who is symptomatic with one caregiver, but it is not known whether the infant/young child is symptomatic with other caregivers, the diagnosis is not to be assigned. Thus, an infant/young child who exhibits chronic food refusal, who has a single caregiver and is not fed by others, would be diagnosed with Undereating Disorder. However, an infant/young child who exhibits food refusal at home with the father, but who eats normally with the caregiver in child care, would qualify for Relationship Specific Disorder of Infancy/Early Childhood rather than Undereating Disorder.

Associated Features Supporting Diagnosis

Axis II ratings regarding the caregiver specified in Relationship Specific Disorder of Infancy/Early Childhood should always be greater than Level 1 when this diagnosis is made. Relationship Specific Disorder of Infancy/Early Childhood may coexist with other Axis I disorders if the symptomatology specified for Relationship Specific Disorder of Infancy/Early Childhood is different from the symptomatology of the other Axis I disorder.

Developmental Features

Symptoms will vary with the age of the infant/young child, but the disorder itself is not different at different ages. Relationship specificity is better documented in infants than in preschool-age young children because preschool-age young children may have internalized relationship patterns and may recreate them in new relationships; therefore, the disorder may be more common in infants than in preschool-age children.

Prevalence

There are no data on the prevalence of this disorder, but in clinical settings, it is seen with some regularity.

Course

The course of this disorder has not been demonstrated, but heterotypic continuity (i.e., when a core developmental dysfunction/impairment continues but the manifestation changes as development progresses) with another Axis I disorder in later childhood is likely.

Risk and Prognostic Features

Infants/young children exhibiting extremes of attachment relationship disturbances are at increased risk for Relationship Specific Disorder of Infancy/Early Childhood. Still, symptomatic behavior and impaired functioning are required for this diagnosis. Because insecure and especially disorganized attachments in infants/young children are associated with increased risk for concurrent and subsequent psychopathology, it is likely that Relationship Specific Disorder of Infancy/Early Childhood increases risk for subsequent Axis I disorders.

Culture-Related Diagnostic Issues

No specific data are available regarding cultural differences, although wide cultural variations in child care practices suggest that this is an important area to explore.

Gender-Related Diagnostic Issues

No specific data are available regarding gender differences.

Differential Diagnosis

This symptomatic behavior of this disorder may appear similar to that of many different Axis I disorders. It is distinguished by the relationship specificity of the symptoms. Impairment must be documented for the diagnosis to be made, which clarifies the difference between this disorder and relationship patterns that are associated only with risk for subsequent maladaptation.

Comorbidity

Comorbidity with other Axis I disorders is possible, but little is known about specific patterns.

Links to DSM–5 and ICD–10

DSM–5: Parent–Child Relational Problem
ICD–10: Other Specified Problems Related to Upbringing (Z62.820)

Axis II
Relational Context

Axis II is used to characterize the infant's/young child's caregiving relationship context. Because of the central importance of the caregiving relationship for development and health in infancy and early childhood, understanding this relationship context should be included in every assessment of infants/young children. Use of this axis facilitates that understanding by encouraging systematic characterization of one or more infant/young child–primary caregiver relationships (Part A) and characterization of the broader caregiving environment, including coparenting, sibling, and other important family relationships that affect the infant's/young child's development (Part B).

In Part A, Table 1 denotes caregiving dimensions, encompassing basic caregiving functions in the primary caregiving relationship, and Table 2 denotes infant/young child contributions to the primary caregiving relationship. In Part B, Table 3 denotes various dimensions of the caregiving environment. By determining whether each of the specific areas listed is a "strength," "not a concern," or a "concern," it is hoped that a clearer picture of the overall relationship context will emerge, as well as areas that may need to be targeted for treatment.

The levels of adaptive functioning in Part A define ranges of relationship adaptation, and in Part B, the levels of adaptive functioning define ranges of qualities of the caregiving environment. That is, each level encompasses a range of functioning rather than a single scale point. The levels are also arranged ordinally, meaning that the four points on the scale are not considered to be equidistant on a continuum. Thus, there is no expectation that each point defines 25% of a population. In fact, Level 1 is expected to encompass all primary caregiving relationships and caregiving environments that do not need clinical attention, which presumably comprise the largest proportion of relationships and caregiving environments in most populations. Level 2 is a risk indicator that may or may not warrant intervention, but Levels 3 and 4 are indicative of clinical levels of disturbances. Also, Relationship Specific Disorder of Early Childhood corresponds to a Level 3 or Level 4 rating on Axis II. However, an Axis II rating of Level 3 or Level 4 does not necessarily imply a relationship specific disorder.

A. CAREGIVER–INFANT/YOUNG CHILD RELATIONSHIP ADAPTATION

This scale is for use by trained infant/young child mental health professionals, in clinical settings, to rate the adaptive quality of the relationship between a primary caregiver and an infant/young child (less than 6 years old). More than one primary caregiving relationship may be the focus of clinical assessment, and separate ratings should be obtained for each primary caregiving relationship assessed. Generally, it is expected that this rating will occur at the conclusion of an assessment process.

The assessment of the parent–infant/young child relationship should, whenever feasible, include observations of parent–infant/young child interactions as well as noting parents' attitudes and attributions about the infant/young child. Observations of interactive behaviors and interviews about caregiver perceptions of the infant/young child each contribute distinctively to a clinical understanding of the relationship. Valid methods exist for the assessment of these two areas using structured instruments, naturalistic observations, and unstructured discussions with caregivers, or a combination of these approaches. Different assessment strategies may be more available and more useful, depending on the clinical circumstances and clinical setting.

Infants/young children typically have a small number of primary caregivers with whom they establish important attachment relationships. The scale is not to be used to rate either caregiver or infant/young child behavior alone but rather the dynamics of the relationship as it exists between the caregiver and infant/young child. The presumption is that disturbances in relationships between infants/young children and their attachment figures may derive from within the caregiver, from within the infant/young child, or from the unique fit between the two.

Although both the caregiver and the infant/young child each individually contribute to the emotional quality of their relationship, the caregiver's effectiveness in providing age-appropriate, sensitive care to the infant/young child is an important influence on the infant's/young child's ability to trust and rely on the caregiver to meet physical and psychological needs. Clinicians may use the caregiving dimensions and the infant/young child contributions described (see Tables 1 and 2) to guide observations and to inform appraisal of the infant/young child–caregiver relationship.

Appraising the adequacy of caregiving requires attention to three overarching characteristics: (1) the caregiver is consistently emotionally available, (2) the caregiver knows and values the infant/young child as a unique individual, and (3) the caregiver is comfortably and competently in charge of raising the infant/young child. Emotional availability requires monitoring the infant/young child, reading cues, and responding effectively. Being in charge effectively overlaps with emotional availability but highlights the importance of setting aside one's own needs sufficiently to be able to meet the needs of the infant/young child. First-time parents with a newborn may need a trial-and-error period of getting to know their infant to develop more confidence and competence, which usually becomes better established as their infant becomes older and communicates his or her needs more clearly. Nevertheless, in healthier relationships, parents adapt to their infant's needs and do not expect the infant to adapt disproportionately to their needs.

Interactions are one important source of information about relationships between infants/young children and caregivers. In addition, the dyad's subjective experience of one another is also an important source of information. Parents and infants/young children are able to convey their subjective experience through verbal and nonverbal behavior.

There is no presumption that the relationship quality between an infant/young child and one primary caregiver is related to the relationship quality between an infant/young child and other primary caregivers. There is considerable evidence that infants/young children may construct different kinds of relationships with different caregivers. The only way to determine the relationship quality between an infant/young child and each specific caregiver is to assess it directly.

Each of the caregiving dimensions listed in Table 1 contributes to the clinician's appraisal of the relationship, but there is no minimum number of concerning dimensions that translates into a specific rating of the level of relationship adaptation.

Specify and describe caregiver and infant/young child contributions to the relationship:

_____

_____

_____

_____

_____

The level chosen represents a summary statement of the overall functioning of the relationship. Each of these levels represents a range from higher to lower functioning rather than a single point. The scale is ordinal rather than continuous, meaning that each level becomes more problematic from 1 to 4, but the levels are not equidistant points on a continuum. Characteristics of the population of caregivers and infants/young children who are being rated will affect the distribution of cases across the different levels. Cultural values, beliefs, and practices of the family should be considered when assigning these ratings. In low-risk populations, Level 1 should predominate.

Table 1. Dimensions of Caregiving

Indicate how each of the caregiving dimensions contributes to relationship quality.

Caregiving Dimension	Contribution to Relationship Quality		
	Strength	*Not a concern*	*Concern*
Ensuring physical safety			
Providing for basic needs (e.g., food, hygiene, clothing, housing, health care)			
Conveying psychological commitment to and emotional investment in the infant/young child			
Establishing structure and routines			
Recognizing and responding to the infant's/young child's emotional needs and signals			
Providing comfort for distress			
Teaching and social stimulation			
Socializing			
Disciplining			
Engaging in play and enjoyable activities			
Showing interest in the infant's/young child's individual experiences and perspectives			
Demonstrating reflective capacity regarding the infant's/young child's developmental trajectory			
Incorporating the infant's/young child's point of view in developmentally appropriate ways			
Tolerating ambivalent feelings in the caregiver–infant/young child relationship			

Find a printable copy of this table on www.zerotothree.org/dc05resources

Table 2. Infant's/Young Child's Contributions to the Relationship

Indicate how each of the infant's/young child's characteristics contributes to relationship quality.

Child Characteristics	Contribution to Relationship Quality		
	Strength	*Not a concern*	*Concern*
Temperamental dispositions			
Sensory profile			
Physical appearance			
Physical health (from Axis III)			
Developmental status (from Axes I and V)			
Mental health (from Axis I)			
Learning style			

Note: Caregiving dimensions and the infant's/young child's characteristics that contribute to relationship quality are inherently culturally bound. Clinicians are encouraged to think carefully about family cultural values and practices that define the infant's/young child's characteristics and which parenting practices are endorsed or proscribed.

Find a printable copy of this table on www.zerotothree.org/dc05resources

Levels of Adaptive Functioning–Caregiving Dimension

The levels that follow indicate the range of functioning that the clinician has determined is the best fit for the relationship in question, on the basis of clinical assessment.

Level 1, *Well-Adapted to Good-Enough Relationships*, describes relationships that are not of clinical concern. This level covers a broad range of relationships, from those that are functioning adequately for both partners on the caregiving dimensions to those that are exemplary. At Level 2, *Strained to Concerning Relationships*, careful monitoring (at least) is definitely indicated, and intervention may be required. At Level 3, *Compromised to Disturbed Relationships*, the relationship disturbance is clearly in the clinical range, and intervention is indicated. Finally, at Level 4, *Disordered to Dangerous Relationships*, intervention is not only required but is urgently needed because of the severity of the relationship impairment. A detailed explanation of each level is presented next:

Level 1—*Well-Adapted to Good-Enough Relationships*

Ratings at this level range from adequate to outstanding infant/young child–caregiver relationships. Ups and downs may be evident, and occasional perturbations may be noted in response to stressors, but the relationship functions adequately or better for both partners most of the time. The infant/young child is consistently protected from danger and shows a prevailing expectation that the caregiver will be reliably available across the different caregiving dimensions. The relationship promotes the infant's/young child's needs for freely expressing emotions and learning to regulate them, for comfort and closeness, and for engaging and exploring. Conflicts are not characteristic of the relationship and are adequately repaired when they occur. In addition, a healthy asymmetry in the relationship is evident in that the caregiver is responsible for the infant's/young child's well-being, but the infant/young child is not responsible for the caregiver's well-being.

Level 2—*Strained to Concerning Relationships*

Relationships show some worrisome patterns of interaction or subjective experience. The relationship is conflicted, insufficiently engaged, or inappropriately imbalanced (e.g., role reversed). Some important adaptive qualities are present. However, there is evidence of a struggle within the relationship or concern about the dyad's capacity for healthy expression of and responding to needs for comfort and protection, or support for and willingness to engage in age-appropriate exploration. There are some limits in mutual enjoyment of activities or expressions of affection and problems in regulation of emotion. Social interactions, including joint play, may not be consistently coordinated, reciprocal, or responsive. There may be some signs of the parent or the infant/young child being insufficiently engaged in interactions. Some interactions may be characterized by unhealthy efforts to control the other. These struggles or concerns extend beyond what is expected in relationships between parents and infants/young children. Parent support services may be indicated.

Level 3—*Compromised to Disturbed Relationships*

Relationships are clearly in the range of clinical concern and require intervention because of risk to the infant's/young child's safety, persistent distress, risk for subsequent problems, or current serious functional impairment. Adaptive qualities may be evident occasionally but are too inconsistent or mostly lacking. There are definite problems with the dyad's emotional communication and social reciprocity that compromise the infant's/young child's emotion regulation. Expressing and responding to needs for comfort and protection, age-appropriate socialization, as well as support for and willingness to engage in play and healthy exploration are impaired. The relationship is fraught with inappropriate levels of risk to safety, significant conflict, insufficient or irregular engagement, or significant imbalance. The level of disturbance indicates that the infant's/young child's social and emotional trajectories have become or are at substantial risk of being compromised.

Level 4—*Disordered to Dangerous Relationships*

Relationships convey an unquestionable urgency about the need to intervene to address serious and potentially dangerous relationship qualities. Not only are adaptive qualities lacking but the relationship pathology is severe and often pervasive, with impairments in the dyad's capacity to engage in adequate protection, emotional availability, and emotion regulation; expressing and responding to needs for comfort and caregiving; as well as support for and willingness to engage in age-appropriate exploration and learning. The relationship may be fraught with significant overt conflict, seriously insufficient engagement much of the time, or significant role reversal. Parental attributions regarding the infant/young child are negative, demonstrate significant developmentally inappropriate expectations, and are not open to reflection or challenge. These disturbances are seriously compromising the infant's/young child's development or may threaten the infant's/young child's physical or psychological safety.

Note: The associations among a disorder in an infant/young child, a disorder in a caregiver, and a disorder in an infant/young child–caregiver relationship are complex. An infant/young child may have a disorder with clinical symptoms and any level of relationship adaptation noted previously, although more impaired relationships are expected when there is a serious Axis I infant/young child diagnosis or severe parental psychopathology. An infant/young child may have an anxiety disorder, Posttraumatic Stress Disorder, or even Autism Spectrum Disorder that is associated with a well-adapted relationship with a primary caregiver, but varying levels of maladaptation are more likely when the infant's/young child's emotional difficulties make caregiving more stressful. Challenging infant/young child behaviors may contribute to and reflect the relationship disturbance. Because infants/young children are especially sensitive to their caregiving environments, relationship maladaptation is likely to increase when parental psychopathology affects the quality of caregiving.

A diagnosis of Relationship Specific Disorder of Infancy/Early Childhood on Axis I corresponds with a Level 3 or 4 rating on Axis II. However, an Axis II rating of Level 3 or 4 does not necessarily imply a relationship specific disorder.

B. CAREGIVING ENVIRONMENT AND INFANT/YOUNG CHILD ADAPTATION

The stability, predictability, and emotional quality of the relationships among the adult caregivers for an infant/young child are important predictors of the infant's/young child's functioning. Infants/young children develop important relationships not only with their primary caregiver(s) but also with other family members, who may either participate in a coparenting relationship with another caregiver or who may affect the infant's/young child's functioning through their influence on the primary caregiver's quality of functioning. Infants/young children are keen observers of how adults who are central in their lives relate to one another and to other people, including other infants/young children in the family or people outside of the family. They often learn by imitation, adopting the behaviors they observe. The affective tone and adult interactions they witness in turn influence the infant's/young child's emotion regulation, trust in relationships, and freedom to explore.

This rating assesses the level of functioning of the *caregiving environment*, defined as the web of caregiving relationships surrounding the infant/young child, regardless of whether the caregivers live together. Because infants/young children construct different relationships with different caregivers, the levels described as follows are meant to indicate the harmoniousness, integration, and coordination among the different caregiving relationships influencing the infant's/young child's functioning. This rating should reflect both the infant's/young child's relationship with different caregivers in the immediate family and the caregivers' cooperative coordination of their goals, values, and behaviors in their care of the infant/young child. Clinicians may use the caregiving dimensions described below to guide their observations and to inform their appraisal of the family caregiving environment and the infant's/young child's adaptation to it.

Data to complete the ratings may be obtained by observations of family and coparent interactions as well as by caregivers' descriptions of the various dimensions listed below. As noted in Part A, both formal and informal methods—each with advantages and disadvantages—may be used.

Table 3. Dimensions of the Caregiving Environment

Indicate how each of the dimensions contributes to the functioning of the caregiving environment.

Caregiving Dimension	Contribution to Relationship Quality		
	Strength	*Not a concern*	*Concern*
Problem solving			
Conflict resolution			
Caregiving role allocation			
Caregiving communication: Instrumental			
Caregiving communication: Emotional			
Emotional investment			
Behavioral regulation and coordination			
Sibling harmony			

Note: Dimensions of the caregiving environment are likely to be understood and defined differently within different cultures and subcultures. Clinicians are encouraged to think carefully about family cultural values and practices and to strike a balance between understanding and accepting cultural variations and intervening with limits that support the infant's/young child's development.

Find a printable copy of this table on www.zerotothree.org/dc05resources

Levels of Adaptive Functioning—Caregiving Environment

The levels that follow indicate the range of functioning that the clinician has determined is the best fit for the caregiving relationship in question, on the basis of clinical assessment. Level 1, *Well-Adapted to Good-Enough Caregiving Environments*, describes caregiving environments that are not of clinical concern. This level covers a broad range of environments, from those that are adequately supportive of the infant's/young child's development to those that are exemplary. At Level 2, *Strained to Concerning Caregiving Environments*, careful monitoring (at least) is definitely indicated, and intervention may be required. At Level 3, *Compromised to Disturbed Caregiving Environments*, the environment is disturbed enough to be considered within the clinical range, and intervention is indicated to address the disturbance. Finally, at Level 4, *Disordered to Dangerous Caregiving Environments*, intervention is not only required but is urgently needed because the effect on the infant's/young child's development is severe. A detailed explanation of each level is presented next:

Level 1—*Well-Adapted to Good-Enough Caregiving Environments*

Relationships at this level range from adequate to outstanding. Ups and downs may be evident, and occasional lapses may occur in response to stressors, but the relationships among the caregivers function adequately or better in their shared care of the infant/young child. The caregivers have a solid repertoire of problem-solving strategies that they generally deploy successfully, and the infant/young child typically shows comfort and ease in interacting with the different caregivers and switching from one to the other according to the demands of the situation. Most of the time, there is a mutually satisfying allocation of caregiving roles and flexibility in mutual support in caring for the infant/young child. The caregivers collaborate adequately with each other in coparenting and meeting the infant's/young child's needs for well-regulated emotions, for comfort and closeness, and for engaging and exploring. Conflicts are not characteristic of the relationship among the caregivers, and the strains that may occur around caregiving priorities and roles are adequately repaired.

Level 2—*Strained to Concerning Caregiving Environments*

Relationships at this level are showing some worrisome patterns of interaction. There are signs of conflict and insufficient communication and coordination among the caregivers regarding the care and upbringing of the infant/young child. The infant/young child experiences distress, tension, or uncertainty about how to negotiate interactions with the different caregivers and may show preferences that spark conflict among them. Some important adaptive qualities are present, but there is also evidence of a struggle within or concern about the caregivers' misalignment of expectations, coordinated emotional availability with the infant/young child, expressing and responding to needs for comfort and protection, age-appropriate socialization, as well as shared support for and willingness to engage in play and exploration. These coparenting struggles or concerns are beginning to extend beyond what is expected in family relationships.

Level 3—*Compromised to Disturbed Caregiving Environments*

Relationships at this level are in the clinical range requiring intervention because of risk to the infant's/young child's safety, persistent distress, risk for subsequent problems, or current serious functional impairment. The caregivers are unable to provide coordinated coparenting or to engage in adaptive problem solving involving the infant/young child. Collaboration and coordination of care may be occasionally evident but are mostly lacking. There are problems with the caregivers' emotional availability (and the infant's/young child's emotion regulation), role allocation, and mutual support in expressing and responding to the infant's/young child's needs for comfort and protection, age-appropriate socialization, as well as support for and willingness to engage in play and exploration. The family relationships are fraught with inappropriate levels of risk to safety, significant conflict, insufficient or irregular engagement, or significant imbalance. The level of disturbance indicates that the infant's/young child's social and emotional trajectories have become or are at risk of being compromised.

Level 4—*Disordered to Dangerous Caregiving Environments*

Relationships at this level convey an unquestionable urgency about intervening to address serious and potentially dangerous relationship conflicts. Not only are adaptive qualities lacking but the relationship pathology among caregivers is severe and pervasive, with significant impairments in the provision of adequate protection and responsive caregiving, age-appropriate socialization, as well as support for exploration and learning. Most of the time, the family relationships are fraught with significant overt conflict, insufficient engagement, or significant role reversal. These disturbances are seriously compromising the infant's/young child's development and threaten the infant's/young child's physical or psychological safety.

Note: In dangerous relationships, when the infant's/young child's safety is threatened, clinicians must consider active interventions to protect the infant/young child, such as a report to child protective services when such services are available or when reports are mandated by local regulations. It should be noted that a rating of Level 4 on the Caregiver–Infant/Young Child Relationship Adaptation or on the Caregiving Environment and Infant/Young Child Adaptation, which on both scales include a range of maladaptive relationships, does not necessarily imply that a mandated report must be made; however, this rating does indicate the need for immediately enhanced caregiving support aimed to protect the infant/young child. Also, relationships that have been characterized by maltreatment in the past should not necessarily receive a Level 4 rating only on the basis of that history if more adaptive qualities are evident during the assessment.

Axis III
Physical Health Conditions and Considerations

Axis III should be used to note physical health conditions and considerations not described in Axis I. A comprehensive, diagnostic assessment includes evaluation of an infant's/young child's physical, cognitive, and developmental conditions in addition to mental health. These health conditions and considerations are generally elicited from medical documentation, family report, or collaboration with the medical provider when risk is identified. The clinical function of the Axis III condition is considered part of a comprehensive formulation. An Axis III condition has a variable influence on mental health status, increasing risk in some instances, promoting resilience in other instances, or at times having no substantial impact.

All aspects of infants'/young children's development are interrelated, and the domains of physical, neurodevelopmental, and mental health overlap and interact substantially. By convention, DC:0–5™ uses Axes I and II to focus on the observable emotional, behavioral, and relational patterns of infants/young children, and Axis III focuses on the physical health conditions. Using this approach, Axis III also includes biological factors or processes that contribute to well-characterized syndromes including Fetal Alcohol Syndrome or Fragile X Syndrome. As our understanding of the complex interactions among biological factors, environmental factors, and psychological processes deepens, it is acknowledged that the distinctions among these categories will likely blur further.

Health conditions may influence mental health directly or indirectly. A health condition, the toxins causing the condition, or the medications used to treat the infant/young child may influence central nervous system functioning through congenital malformations, injuries, or insults. In addition., the experience of physical symptoms—including pain, itching, or respiratory distress—may affect emotional expression, sleep, and feeding patterns. Axis III includes specific attention to pregnancy and perinatal complications that can have direct influences on the infant's/young child's development. Indirectly, medical conditions may influence an infant's/young child's experiences by exposure to potentially traumatic medical procedures (even when they are lifesaving) and through the limitations on normative activities and interactions because of physical disabilities, fragile immune status, or schedule. Chronic or acute medical conditions may result in separations from primary caregivers and exposure to a high number of health caregivers and, thus, may influence the functioning of the family through fatigue, financial stressors, stress, and related means. Psychologically, health conditions often influence a parent's perception of the infant's/young child's vulnerability or resilience as well as the infant's/young child's perception of him- or herself, especially in the case of visible congenital malformations or chronic medical illnesses. The attribution of responsibility for the medical condition may also influence family interactions. It should be noted that indirect influences may be neutral, promote resilience, or amplify risk.

As evidence of the complex interactions among physical health, caregiving environment, and mental health, some health conditions may also reflect characteristics of the caregiving environment, such as prenatal exposure to alcohol or injuries sustained through maltreatment.

Historical health conditions have the potential to influence the parent–infant/young child relationship and may play a role in the infant's/young child's mental health and development long after the medical condition has resolved. For this reason, Axis III is considered inclusive of all health conditions that could influence the clinical presentation, not just those conditions about which the clinician has absolute certainty.

Awareness of the diagnosis is more important than technical accuracy. Parents may describe medical illnesses in terms that do not provide medical specificity of the condition; however, their descriptions should also be noted under Axis III (e.g., "hole in heart"), and clarifying information may subsequently be obtained from pediatric providers.

The categories described in our examples below include prenatal medical conditions, chronic medical conditions, acute medical conditions, medical procedures, pain, physical indicators of caregiving environment problems, medications, and markers of health status. These categories are not mutually exclusive, and a condition should only be listed once in the diagnosis. The health domains are representative of some areas of health that should be considered, but the list is not exhaustive, and all areas identified in the clinical assessment should be included under Axis III:

- **Prenatal conditions and exposures**
  - Exposure to medications or substances that may include but are not limited to fetal alcohol and other substance exposure, environmental teratogen exposure, or prenatal medication exposure
  - Prematurity
  - Prenatally identified medical conditions (e.g., congenital malformations or genetic abnormalities)

- **Chronic medical conditions**
  - Allergies (e.g., eczema, chronic ear infections, or food and environmental allergies)
  - Colic
  - Congenital anomalies (e.g., cardiac, facial, limb, and others)
  - Cancers and tumors

- Endocrine (e.g., thyroid, growth hormone deficiencies or exogenous use of hormone replacement, diabetes, congenital adrenal hyperplasia, and other causes of ambiguous genitalia)
- Gastrointestinal (e.g., reflux, constipation, diarrhea, or medical or elective diet restrictions such as a gluten-free diet)
- Growth trajectory problems (e.g., nutritional insufficiency, failure to thrive, small head circumference, short stature, or obesity)
- Genetic syndromes (e.g., Down syndrome, DiGeorge syndrome, Turner syndrome, Fragile X syndrome, or Williams syndrome)
- Hematologic and blood diseases (e.g., hemophilia, anemia, or sickle cell disease)
- Immunization status
- Neurologic conditions (e.g., seizure disorders, hydrocephalus, or intra-ventricular hemorrhage)
- Metabolic conditions (e.g., storage diseases, mitochondrial disorders, or urea cycle disorders)
- Immunologic (e.g., autoimmune disorders [including systemic lupus erythematosus, juvenile rheumatoid arthritis, and hyperthyroidism], central nervous system infections or inflammation, or encephalopathies [including Pediatric Autoimmune Neuropsychiatric Disorders Associated with Streptococcal Infections and post-infectious encephalopathies])
- Infectious disease (e.g., HIV/AIDS, polio, tuberculosis, measles, and many others)
- Respiratory (e.g., asthma or cystic fibrosis)
- Sensory problems (e.g., vision or hearing impairment)
- Dental (e.g., caries or fractures)

- **Acute medical conditions** (e.g., trauma, accidents, fractures, appendicitis, or acute infections)

- **History of procedures** (regardless of final diagnosis)

- **Recurrent or chronic pain** (from any cause)

- **Physical injuries or exposures reflective of the caregiving environment** (e.g., bruises, burns, or other injuries; injuries related to sexual abuse; or accidental chemical or medication ingestions)

- **Medication effects** (e.g., steroids, albuterol, antihistamines, pain medications, anti-epileptic medications, psychotropic medications, or over-the-counter dietary supplements)

- **Markers of health status** (identified through primary care and dental providers as well as immunization status)

Note: Excessive Crying Disorder (colic) should be coded under Axis I; however, co-occurring conditions, such as a diagnosis of gastroesophageal reflux, can be included under Axis III.

Axis IV
Psychosocial Stressors

Axis IV provides a framework for identifying and evaluating psychosocial and environmental stressors that may influence the presentation, course, treatment, and prevention of mental health symptoms and disorders in infants/young children. Research indicates that for many infants/young children, stressors often co-occur. The *cumulative risk hypothesis*, which has increasing empirical support, suggests that the number of stressors is more predictive of subsequent maladaptation than any specific stressors. The consequence of this hypothesis is that a comprehensive consideration of stressors affecting the infant/young child is an important part of understanding an infant/young child in context.

Psychosocial stressors for an infant/young child include acute events and enduring circumstances. Examples of the latter include poverty and domestic violence. Moreover, stress may be direct (e.g., an illness requiring the infant's/young child's hospitalization) or indirect (e.g., a sudden illness of a parent). Even events and transitions that are part of normal experience in the family's culture, nevertheless, may be stressful for an infant/young child—for example, the birth of a sibling, a family move, a parent returning to work after being at home, or entry into child care. Some infants/young children will experience these transitions as stressful, whereas others make transitions smoothly and adapt to new circumstances easily.

The caregiving environment may shield and protect the infant/young child from stressful events and circumstances, thereby lessening their impact. However, caregivers themselves, and their responses to stressful events, are negatively affected by the same stressors. Ultimately, the impact of a stressful event or enduring circumstance depends largely on three factors:

1. The severity of the stressor (its intensity, duration, and predictability).

2. The developmental level of the infant/young child.

3. The availability and capacity of adults in the caregiving environment to serve as protective buffers and to help the infant/young child understand and cope with the stressor.

PSYCHOSOCIAL AND ENVIRONMENTAL STRESSORS FOR THE IDENTIFIED INFANT/YOUNG CHILD

This list provides the clinician with a framework for (1) identifying the multiple sources of stress experienced by an individual infant/young child and family and (2) noting their duration and severity. Note: the items listed in each category are examples and the list is not exhaustive.

To capture the cumulative severity of stressors, the clinician should identify all the sources of stress in an infant's/young child's circumstances. For example, an infant/young child who enters foster placement may be experiencing the impact of abuse, parental psychiatric illness, separation, and poverty. The greater the number of stressors involved, the greater the adverse impact on the infant/young child is presumed to be.

Find a printable copy of this table on www.zerotothree.org/dc05resources

Table 4. Psychosocial and Environmental Stressors

(Complete information for all stressors that apply)

Stressors	Age of onset *(in months)*	Comments, including duration and severity
Challenges within the infant's/young child's family or primary support group		
Acculturation or language conflicts		
Birth of a sibling		
Change in primary caregiver		
Criminal activity within the household		
Death of a parent or important caregiver		
Death of another important person		
Death of other family member		
Domestic violence		
Emotional abuse		
Family social isolation		

Stressors	Age of onset (in months)	Comments, including duration and severity
Father or mother absence		
Inadequate social support for the family		
Incarceration of family member		
Infant/young child has been adopted		
Infant/young child neglect		
Infant/young child physical abuse		
Infant/young child placed in foster care		
Infant/young child placed in institutional care		
Infant/young child reunification with parent after prolonged separation		
Infant/young child sexual abuse		
Medical illness of parent or caregiver (specify acute or chronic)		
Medical illness of sibling or other household member (specify acute or chronic)		
Mental health problems of household member		
New adult in household (e.g., romantic partner)		
New infant/young child (not by birth) in home (e.g., adoption, stepsibling, foster child)		
Other trauma to significant person in the infant/young child's life		
Parent or caregiver discord or conflict (nonphysical)		
Parent or caregiver divorce or separation		
Parent or caregiver mental health problems		
Parent or caregiver remarriage		

Stressors	Age of onset *(in months)*	Comments, including duration and severity
Parent or caregiver separation from the infant/young child (e.g., out-of-town employment, hospitalization)		
Parent or caregiver substance abuse		
Removal of nonindex infant/young child from home		
Severe discord or violence with sibling		
Substance abuse by household member		
Teenage parent		
Unpredictable home environment		
Unstable family constellation		
Challenges in the social environment		
Discrimination or racism is experienced by family		
Immigrant status		
Inadequate access to health care		
Infant/young child experiences bullying		
Infant/young child is witness to community violence		
Refugee status		
Unsafe neighborhood		
Educational or child care challenges		
Multiple changes in child care provider		
Parent or caregiver low literacy		
Poor quality early learning environment or out-of-home care (e.g., health and safety concerns, high infant/young child–staff ratios and large groups, inadequately trained staff, lack of attention to social and emotional development)		

Stressors	Age of onset *(in months)*	Comments, including duration and severity
Housing challenges		
Eviction from home or foreclosure		
Homelessness		
Inadequate, unsafe, or overcrowded housing		
Multiple moves		
Economic and employment challenges		
Dangerous or stressful parental work conditions		
Food insecurity		
Heavy indebtedness		
Military deployment or reintegration		
Parental unemployment or job instability		
Poverty or near poverty		
Infant/young child health		
Infant/young child accident or injury (e.g., animal bite, passenger in vehicular accident)		
Infant/young child hospitalization		
Infant/young child medical illness (acute or chronic)		
Painful or frightening medical procedure(s)		
Pregnancy-related stressors		
Legal or criminal justice challenges		
Child protective services involvement		
Custody dispute		
Infant/young child is victim of crime		

Stressors	Age of onset *(in months)*	Comments, including duration and severity
Parent is victim of crime		
Parental arrest		
Parental deportation		
Parental incarceration or return from incarceration		
Undocumented immigration status		
Other		
Abduction (specify by family member or nonfamily member)		
Disaster (e.g., fire, hurricane, earthquake)		
Disease epidemic		
Terrorism		
War		
Other (specify)		

Note: "Parent" refers to parenting figure(s).

Axis V
Developmental Competence

Axis V uses an integrative model for understanding the infant's/young child's developmental competencies in the domains of emotional, social-relational, language-social communication, cognitive, as well as movement and physical development. The information in Axis V may be used to examine how developmental domains function together (not discreetly) and within the context of the other axes to inform the diagnostic process. Axis V is included because infant/young child mental health can only be understood within the context of developmental competencies, which emerge in an integrated fashion within interactions with important caregivers.

Emotional and social capacities are present at birth, and these competencies serve as the foundation for all development. Understanding the manner in which the infant/young child integrates competencies in and across different developmental domains is necessary for clinical formulation that highlights the infant's/young child's demonstrated capacities within and across emotional, social, and relational domains. The infant/young child makes use of earlier capacities to reach higher levels of functioning. Axis V was designed to provide the clinician with a more comprehensive understanding of the infant's/young child's developmental profile to inform clinical and diagnostic formulations.

Developmental Competence: These ratings can be informed by observations of the infant's/young child's interactions with caregivers and toys, parent reports, results of developmental screening tools, standard scores based on formal developmental testing, or the developmental milestones chart presented in Appendix A: Developmental Milestones and Competency Ratings. The developmental milestones included in Appendix A can serve as guides and can aid in anchoring an infant's/young child's developmental capacities but are not presented as a replacement for other modes of assessment.

COMPETENCY DOMAIN RATING SUMMARY TABLE

On the basis of the review of this infant's/young child's developmental capacities, complete the table below to indicate the category that best describes the infant's/young child's functioning in each of the domains that comprise Axis V:

To be completed for all infants/young children. Indicate competency domain rating scores by placing an "X" in the box for the appropriate score for each developmental domain.

Find a printable copy of this table on www.zerotothree.org/dc05resources

Competency Domain Rating	Emotional	Social-Relational	Language-Social Communication	Cognitive	Movement and Physical
Exceeds developmental expectations					
Functions at age-appropriate level					
Competencies are inconsistently present or emerging					
Not meeting developmental expectations (delay or deviance)					

Overall impression. Provide Axis V formulation as an overall impression on the basis of the ratings above. Indicate any unevenness of developmental competencies highlighting relative strengths and concerns. Also note whether there have been any recent changes in competencies in any developmental domain.

_____

_____

_____

_____

_____

Appendix A
Developmental Milestones and Competency Ratings

When using the table provided in this appendix, the clinician should begin with the age-expected capacities of the infant/young child. If the infant/young child is not meeting age-expected capacities in any domain, the clinician should keep assessing at developmentally earlier categories. It is important to rate the infant's/young child's functioning in each of the domains (i.e., emotional, social-relational, language-social communication, cognitive, and movement and physical development) as well as to note consistencies and inconsistencies within and across domains of developmental functioning. To complete the chart, first rate how the infant/young child is developing in each of the listed domains using the rating scale that is presented below. Indicate a rating for each milestone included in the domain and then conclude with a representative domain rating based on the pattern of individual milestones for each domain. To complete Axis V, review the pattern of ratings across domains to determine an overall rating for the infant/young child.

Note: This table represents samples of key milestones gathered from a variety of established sources and is a representative, but not exhaustive, listing for the clinician's reference. It is intended to be used as a way to document observations about an infant's/young child's developmental functioning. It is not a substitute for a standardized, validated developmental assessment. The milestone chart is organized both by domain and infant/young child age. We prioritize behaviors that one would expect to observe within the specified developmental periods. For sources of developmental capacities, please refer to the reference list at the end of this appendix.

Rate individual behaviors in the age or mental age range as follows:

1 = Fully present

2 = Inconsistently present or emerging

3 = Absent

Find a printable copy of these tables on www.zerotothree.org/dc05resources

By 3 months old

Competency Domain	Milestone	Milestone Rating	Comments	Competency Domain Rating
Emotional	Briefly calms self (e.g., sucks on hand).			
	Exhibits interest in the outside world when in an alert state (e.g., gazes at objects, people, or light; localizes to sound; adjusts breathing in response to sound of voices).			
	Is comforted by proximity to caregiver and soothing motion.			
	Remains in a calm, focused state for at least 2 minutes.			
	Makes smooth state transitions (e.g., sleep to drowsy to awake).			
	Expresses contentment or discomfort.			
Social-Relational	Smiles responsively (i.e., social smile).			
	Looks at caregiver's face.			
	Coos responsively.			
	Localizes to familiar voices and sounds.			
	Shows interest in facial expressions.			
Language-Social Communication	Follows sounds (e.g., turning head in response to sound).			
	Coos and gurgles.			
	Imitates simple facial expressions (e.g., smiling, sticking tongue out).			

Rating key: 1 = Fully present; 2 = Inconsistently present or emerging; 3 = Absent.

By 3 months old

Competency Domain	Milestone	Milestone Rating	Comments	Competency Domain Rating
Cognitive	Follows people and objects with eyes.			
	Loses interest or protests if activity does not change.			
Movement and Physical	Pushes up trunk when lying on stomach.			
	Holds head up without support.			
	Hands are often open (i.e., not in fists).			

Rating key: 1 = Fully present; 2 = Inconsistently present or emerging; 3 = Absent.

By 6 months old

Competency Domain	Milestone	Milestone Rating	Comments	Competency Domain Rating
Emotional	Responds to affection with smiling, cooing, or settling.			
	Demonstrates a range of emotions that includes happiness, excitement, sadness, fear, distress, disgust, anger, joy, interest, and surprise.			
	Expresses anger, frustration, or protest with distinct cries and facial expressions.			
	Recovers from distress when comforted by caregiver.			
Social-Relational	Imitates some movements and facial expressions (e.g., smiling or frowning).			
	Engages in socially reciprocal interactions (e.g., playing simple back-and-forth games).			
	Seeks social engagement with vocalizations, emotional expressions, or physical contact.			
	Watches faces closely.			
Language-Social Communication	Copies sounds.			
	Babbles with *p*, *b*, and *m* sounds.			
	Vocalizes excitement and displeasure (e.g., laughs and coos).			
	Produces distinct cries to show hunger, pain, or being tired.			

Rating key: 1 = Fully present; 2 = Inconsistently present or emerging; 3 = Absent.

By 6 months old

Competency Domain	Milestone	Milestone Rating	Comments	Competency Domain Rating
Cognitive	Tracks moving objects with eyes from side to side.			
	Experiments with cause and effect (e.g., bangs spoon on table).			
	Smiles and vocalizes in response to own face in mirror image.			
	Recognizes familiar people and things at a distance.			
	Demonstrates anticipation of certain routine activities (e.g., shows excitement in anticipation of being fed).			
Movement and Physical	Swats at dangling objects.			
	Pushes down on legs when feet are on a hard surface.			
	Sits without support.			
	Rolls over from tummy to back.			
	Holds and shakes an object.			
	Bangs two objects together.			
	Brings hands to midline.			
	Reaches for object with one hand.			

Rating key: 1 = Fully present; 2 = Inconsistently present or emerging; 3 = Absent.

By 9 months old

Competency Domain	Milestone	Milestone Rating	Comments	Competency Domain Rating
Emotional	Has strategies for self-soothing.			
	Demonstrates preference for caregivers.			
	Intentionally communicates feelings to others.			
Social-Relational	Distinguishes between familiar and unfamiliar voices.			
	Shows some stranger wariness.			
	Protests separation from caregiver.			
	Enjoys extended play with others, especially caregivers.			
	Engages in back-and-forth, two-way communication using vocalizations and eye contact.			
	Mimics other's simple gestures.			
	Follows other's gaze and pointing.			
Language-Social Communication	Responds to sounds by making sounds or moving body.			
	Imitates speech sounds when prompted			
	Begins to use noncrying sounds (speech sounds) to get and keep attention			
	String vowels together when babbling (*ah, eh, oh*).			
	Makes sounds to show joy or displeasure			

Rating key: 1 = Fully present; 2 = Inconsistently present or emerging; 3 = Absent.

By 9 months old

Competency Domain	Milestone	Milestone Rating	Comments	Competency Domain Rating
Language-Social Communication	Begins to use gestures to communicate wants and needs (e.g., reaches to be picked up).			
	Follows some routine commands when paired with gestures			
	Shows understanding of commonly used words.			
Cognitive	Mouths or bangs objects.			
	Tries to get objects that are out of reach.			
	Looks for things he or she sees others hide (e.g., toy under blanket).			
Movement and Physical	Rolls over in both directions (front to back, back to front).			
	Brings self to sitting position independently.			
	Stands with support.			
	Moves independently from one place to another (e.g., crawling, scooting).			
	Turns pages of a book.			
	Reaches for and grasps objects.			
	Passes objects from one hand to the other.			

Rating key: 1 = Fully present; 2 = Inconsistently present or emerging; 3 = Absent.

By 12 months old

Competency Domain	Milestone	Milestone Rating	Comments	Competency Domain Rating
Emotional	Looks to caregiver for information about new situations and environments.			
	Looks to caregiver to share emotional experiences.			
	Responds to other people's emotions (e.g., displays sober, serious face in response to sadness in parent; smiles when parent laughs).			
	Uses gestures to communicate feelings (e.g., clapping when excited).			
Social-Relational	Offers object to initiate interaction (e.g., hands caregiver a book to hear a story).			
	Plays interactive games (e.g., "peek-a-boo" and "pat-a-cake").			
	Looks at familiar people when they are named.			
	Gives object to seek help (e.g., hands shoe to parent).			
	Extends arm or leg to assist with dressing.			
Language-Social Communication	Understands "no."			
	Responds to own name.			
	Looks in response to "where" questions (e.g., "Where is the doggie?").			
	Makes different consonant sounds such as *mamamam* and *babababa*.			
	Points to nearby objects.			
	Imitates conventional gestures (e.g., waving bye-bye, clapping).			

Rating key: 1 = Fully present; 2 = Inconsistently present or emerging; 3 = Absent.

By 12 months old

Competency Domain	Milestone	Milestone Rating	Comments	Competency Domain Rating
Language-Social Communication	Responds to simple directives accompanied by gestures such as "come here."			
	Has a few words (e.g., "mama," "dada," "hi," "bye-bye," or "dog").			
Cognitive	Watches the path of something as it falls.			
	Has favorite objects (e.g., toys, blanket).			
	Explores objects and how they work in multiple ways (e.g., mouthing, touching, dropping).			
	Fills and dumps containers.			
	Plays with two objects at the same time.			
Movement and Physical	Takes a few steps without holding on.			
	Walks holding onto furniture (i.e., cruises).			
	Moves from sitting to standing position.			
	Stands alone.			
	Picks up things between thumb and index finger (e.g., cereal).			
	Crawls forward on belly, pulling with arms and pushing with legs.			
	Turns around while crawling.			
	Crawls while holding an object.			

Rating key: 1 = Fully present; 2 = Inconsistently present or emerging; 3 = Absent.

By 15 months old

Competency Domain	Milestone	Milestone Rating	Comments	Competency Domain Rating
Emotional	Shows affection with kisses (without pursed lips).			
	Demonstrates cautious or fearful behavior such as clinging to or hiding behind caregiver.			
Social-Relational	Seeks and enjoys attention from others, especially caregivers.			
	Engages in parallel play with peers.			
	Presents a book or toy when he or she wants to hear a story or to play.			
	Repeats sounds or actions to get attention.			
	Enjoys looking at picture books with caregiver.			
Language-Social Communication	Uses simple gestures such as shaking head "no" or waving "bye-bye."			
	Responds to the gestures of others.			
	Enjoys looking at picture books with caregivers.			
	Makes sounds with changes in tone (sounds more like speech).			
	Uses complex communication skills integrating gestures, vocalizations, and eye contact (e.g., looking to parent while taking his or her hand to bring him or her to a desired toy).			

Rating key: 1 = Fully present; 2 = Inconsistently present or emerging; 3 = Absent.

By 15 months old

Competency Domain	Milestone	Milestone Rating	Comments	Competency Domain Rating
Language-Social Communication	Identifies correct picture or object when it is named.			
	Follows simple requests (e.g., "pick up the toy"; "roll the ball").			
Cognitive	Imitates complex gestures (e.g., signing).			
	Initiates joint attention (e.g., points to show others something interesting or to get others' attention).			
	Finds hidden objects easily.			
	Uses objects for their intended purpose (e.g., drinks from a cup, smooths hair with brush).			
Movement and Physical	Explores physical environment.			
	Pushes objects (e.g., boxes, toy trucks, push toys).			
	Walks independently.			

Rating key: 1 = Fully present; 2 = Inconsistently present or emerging; 3 = Absent.

By 18 months old

Competency Domain	Milestone	Milestone Rating	Comments	Competency Domain Rating
Emotional	Demonstrates self-comforting strategies.			
	Shares humor with peers or adults (e.g., laughs at and makes funny faces or non-sense rhymes).			
Social-Relational	Likes to hand things to others during play.			
	Engages in reciprocal displays of affection (e.g., hugs or kisses with a pucker).			
	Asserts autonomy (e.g., "me do").			
	Reacts with concern when someone appears hurt.			
	Leaves caregiver's side to explore nearby objects or setting.			
	Engages in teasing behavior such as looking at parent and caregiver and doing something "forbidden."			
Language-Social Communication	Uses at least 20 words or word approximations such as *baba* for ball.			
	Shows consistent increases in vocabulary each month.			
	Says and shakes head "no."			
	Can follow one-step verbal commands without any gestures (e.g., sits when you say "sit down").			
	When pointing, looks back to caregiver to confirm joint attention.			
	Combines words, gestures, and eye contact to communicate feelings and requests.			

Rating key: 1 = Fully present; 2 = Inconsistently present or emerging; 3 = Absent.

By 18 months old

Competency Domain	Milestone	Milestone Rating	Comments	Competency Domain Rating
Cognitive	Enacts play sequences with objects according to their intended use (e.g., pushing a toy dump truck and empty-ing its cargo).			
	Shows interest in a doll or stuffed animal by giving a hug.			
	Points to at least one body part.			
	Points to self when asked.			
	Plays simple pretend games (e.g., feeding a doll).			
	Scribbles with crayon, marker, and so forth.			
	Turns pages of book.			
	Recognizes self in mirror.			
Movement and Physical	Stacks two blocks.			
	Walks up steps with help.			
	Pulls toys while walking.			
	Helps undress him- or her-self (e.g., pulls off hat, socks, mittens).			
	Eats with a spoon.			
	Drinks from open cup.			

Rating key: 1 = Fully present; 2 = Inconsistently present or emerging; 3 = Absent.

By 24 months old

Competency Domain	Milestone	Milestone Rating	Comments	Competency Domain Rating
Emotional	Exhibits embarrassment and pride.			
	Exhibits shame and guilt.			
	Exhibits empathy (e.g., offers comfort when someone is hurt).			
	Attempts to exert independence frequently.			
	Names or understands words for basic emotions.			
Social-Relational	Imitates others' complex actions, especially adults and older children (e.g., putting plates on the table, posture, gestures).			
	Enjoys being with other young children.			
	Takes pride and pleasure in independent accomplishments.			
	Primarily plays in proximity to other young children but notices and imitates other young children's play more frequently.			
	Responds to being corrected or praised.			
Language-Social Communication	Enjoys being read to.			
	Names actions.			
	Knows names of familiar people and many body parts.			
	Uses two words together (e.g., "more cookie"; "Dada, bye-bye?").			
	Repeats words overheard in conversation.			

Rating key: 1 = Fully present; 2 = Inconsistently present or emerging; 3 = Absent.

By 24 months old

Competency Domain	Milestone	Milestone Rating	Comments	Competency Domain Rating
Language-Social Communication	Names objects in picture books (e.g., cat, bird, ball, or dog).			
	Imitates animal sounds such as "meow," "woof," "baa," and "moo."			
	Uses some self-referential pronouns such as "mine."			
Cognitive	Finds things even when hidden under two or three covers or when hidden in one place and moved to a second place (i.e., does not give up when the hidden object is not in the first location).			
	Begins to sort shapes and colors.			
	Completes sentences and rhymes from familiar books, stories, or songs.			
	Plays simple make-believe games (e.g., pretend meal).			
	Builds towers of four or more blocks.			
	Follows two-step instructions (e.g., "Pick up your shoes and put them in the closet").			
Movement and Physical	Participates in dressing (e.g., putting arms into sleeves, pulling pants up or down, putting on hat).			
	Stands on tiptoes.			
	Kicks a ball.			
	Runs.			
	Climbs onto and down from furniture without help.			

Rating key: 1 = Fully present; 2 = Inconsistently present or emerging; 3 = Absent.

By 24 months old

Competency Domain	Milestone	Milestone Rating	Comments	Competency Domain Rating
Movement and Physical	Walks up and down stairs holding on.			
	Draws lines.			
	Drinks using a straw.			
	Opens cabinets, drawers, and boxes.			

Rating key: 1 = Fully present; 2 = Inconsistently present or emerging; 3 = Absent.

By 36 months old

Competency Domain	Milestone	Milestone Rating	Comments	Competency Domain Rating
Emotional	Expresses full range of emotions, including pride, shame, guilt, and empathy.			
	Expresses distress or anger with words.			
	Shows pride in new learning and new experiences.			
	Expresses affection openly and verbally.			
	Expresses feelings through pretend play and drama.			
Social-Relational	Shows affection to peers without prompting.			
	Shares without prompts.			
	Can wait turn in playing games.			
	Shows concern for crying peer by taking action.			
	Engages in associative play with peers (i.e., infants/ young children participate in similar activities without formal organization but with some interaction).			
	Shares accomplishments with others.			
	Helps with simple household tasks.			
Language-Social Communication	Clearly uses *k, g, f, t, d,* and *n* sounds.			
	Builds logical bridges between ideas using words such as "but" and "because."			
	Asks questions using words such as "why?" or "how?"			
	Says first name when asked.			

Rating key: 1 = Fully present; 2 = Inconsistently present or emerging; 3 = Absent.

By 36 months old

Competency Domain	Milestone	Milestone Rating	Comments	Competency Domain Rating
Language-Social Communication	Names most familiar objects.			
	Understands words such as "in," "on," and "under."			
	Knows own identifying information (e.g., name, age, gender).			
	Identifies peers by name.			
	Uses some plurals (e.g., "cars," "dogs," "cats").			
	Uses labels "mine," "I," "you," "me," "their," "his," or "hers" accurately.			
	Speaks well enough for familiar listeners to understand most of the time.			
	Carries on a conversation using two or three sentences.			
	Uses sentences that are at least three to four words.			
Cognitive	Labels some colors correctly.			
	Plays thematic make-believe with objects, animals, and people.			
	Answers simple "why" questions (e.g., "Why do we need a coat when it's cold outside?").			
	Shows awareness of skill limitations.			
	Understands "bigger" and "smaller."			
	Understands concept of "two."			
	Enacts complex behavioral routines observed in daily life of caregivers, siblings, or peers.			

Rating key: 1 = Fully present; 2 = Inconsistently present or emerging; 3 = Absent.

By 36 months old

Competency Domain	Milestone	Milestone Rating	Comments	Competency Domain Rating
Cognitive	Solves simple problems (e.g., obtains a desired object by opening a container).			
	Attends to a story for 5 minutes.			
	Plays independently for 5 minutes.			
Movement and Physical	Manipulates some buttons, levers, and moving parts.			
	Climbs on high and low structures.			
	Runs fluidly.			
	Copies a circle.			
	Builds tower of more than six blocks.			
	Pedals a tricycle (three-wheel bicycle).			
	Catches and kicks big ball.			
	Walks up and down steps, alternating feet.			

Rating key: 1 = Fully present; 2 = Inconsistently present or emerging; 3 = Absent.

By 48 months old

Competency Domain	Milestone	Milestone Rating	Comments	Competency Domain Rating
Emotional	Expresses distress or anger with words.			
	Conveys emotional experiences in pretend play.			
	Complies with basic cultural rules for emotional expression.			
Social-Relational	Pretends to play "Mom" and "Dad" (or other relevant caregivers).			
	Asks about or talks about parent and caregiver when separated (i.e., holds the other in mind).			
	Engages in cooperative play with other infants/young children.			
	Has a preferred friend.			
	Expresses interests, likes, and dislikes.			
Language-Social Communication	Relates experiences from school or outside home.			
	Describes events or things using four or more sentences at a time.			
	Identifies rhyming words such as "cat–hat" or "ping–ring."			
	Recognizes and understands basic rules of grammar (e.g., plurals, tense).			
	Sings a song or says a poem from memory (e.g., "Itsy Bitsy Spider" or the "Wheels on the Bus").			
	Tells stories.			
	Says first and last name when asked.			

Rating key: 1 = Fully present; 2 = Inconsistently present or emerging; 3 = Absent.

By 48 months old

Competency Domain	Milestone	Milestone Rating	Comments	Competency Domain Rating
Language-Social Communication	Uses words or adjectives to describe or talk about him- or herself.			
	Understands, uses, and responds to questions of "how" or "when."			
	Uses words that talk about time.			
	Speech is generally understood by nonfamily members.			
Cognitive	Names several colors and some numbers.			
	Counts to five.			
	Has rudimentary understanding of time.			
	Shares past experiences.			
	Remembers parts of a story.			
	Engages in make-believe play with capacity to build and elaborate on play themes.			
	Connects actions and emotions.			
	Responds to questions that require understanding the idea of "same" and "different."			
	Draws a person with two to four body parts.			
	Understands that actions can influence others' emotions (e.g., tries to make others laugh by telling simple jokes).			
	Waits for turn in simple games.			

Rating key: 1 = Fully present; 2 = Inconsistently present or emerging; 3 = Absent.

By 48 months old

Competency Domain	Milestone	Milestone Rating	Comments	Competency Domain Rating
Cognitive	Elaborates on thematic make-believe play.			
	Plays board or card games with simple rules.			
	Describes what is going to happen next in a book.			
	Talks about right and wrong.			
Movement and Physical	Skips, hops, and stands on one foot for up to 2 seconds.			
	Catches a large, bounced ball most of the time.			
	Copies "plus" sign.			
	Uses toilet during the day with few accidents.			
	Pours from one container to another, cuts with supervision, and mashes own food.			

Rating key: 1 = Fully present; 2 = Inconsistently present or emerging; 3 = Absent.

By 60 months old

Competency Domain	Milestone	Milestone Rating	Comments	Competency Domain Rating
Emotional	Expresses two or more emotions at the same time.			
	Shows awareness of and interest in personal success.			
	Shows increased confidence associated with greater independence and autonomy.			
Social-Relational	Wants to please friends.			
	Emulates role models, real or imaginary.			
	Values rules in social interactions.			
	Participates in group activities that require assuming roles (e.g., Follow the Leader).			
	Modulates or modifies voice correctly depending on situation or listener (e.g., outside voice, to adult, other infant/ young child, or younger child).			
Language-Social Communication	Makes all speech sounds. May make mistakes on more difficult sounds such as *ch*, *sh*, *th*, *l*, *v*, and *z* (linguistically variable).			
	Understands words denoting order such as "first," "second," "third," "next," and "last."			
	Uses "today," "yesterday," "tomorrow," "last week," and "before" correctly.			
	Discriminates rhyming and nonrhyming words.			
	Recognizes words with same beginning sound.			

Rating key: 1 = Fully present; 2 = Inconsistently present or emerging; 3 = Absent.

By 60 months old

Competency Domain	Milestone	Milestone Rating	Comments	Competency Domain Rating
Language-Social Communication	Identifies individual sounds within words (e.g., "dog": d–o–g).			
	Tells a simple story using full sentences.			
	Uses future tense (e.g., "Grandma will be here").			
	Says full name and address.			
Cognitive	Counts 10 or more things.			
	Tells stories with beginning, middle, and conclusion.			
	Draws a person with at least six body parts.			
	Acknowledges own mistakes or misbehaviors and can apologize.			
	Distinguishes fantasy from reality most of the time.			
	Names four colors correctly.			
	Follows rules in simple games.			
	Knows function of everyday household objects (e.g., money, cooking utensils, appliances).			
	Attends to group activity for 15 minutes (e.g., circle time, storytelling).			
Movement and Physical	Stands on one foot for 10 seconds or longer.			
	Copies a triangle and other geometric shapes.			
	Copies some letters or numbers.			
	Hops on one foot.			

Rating key: 1 = Fully present; 2 = Inconsistently present or emerging; 3 = Absent.

By 60 months old

Competency Domain	Milestone	Milestone Rating	Comments	Competency Domain Rating
Movement and Physical	Uses utensils to eat.			
	Uses the toilet independently (wipes, flushes, and washes hands).			
	Swings independently on a swing.			

Rating key: 1 = Fully present; 2 = Inconsistently present or emerging; 3 = Absent.

Appendix B
The Process of Revising and Updating DC:0–3R

Revising and Updating DC:0–3R

A 3-year plan for carrying out the revision and update of the *Diagnostic Classification of Mental Health and Developmental Disorders of Infancy and Early Childhood, Revised Edition* (DC:0–3R; ZERO TO THREE, 2005) was presented to and approved by the Executive Committee of ZERO TO THREE in January 2013. The plan included the following: a survey of DC:0–3R users, a review of clinical literature, drafting and eliciting comments on draft criteria, and additional communication with world-renowned clinical experts in particular areas of diagnosis and treatment. The plan also included connecting with various organizations—American Academy of Pediatrics, American Psychological Association, International Association for Child and Adolescent Psychiatry and Allied Professions, International Society for Traumatic Stress Studies, American Occupational Therapy Association, National Child Traumatic Stress Network, American Academy of Child and Adolescent Psychiatry, and Society for Research in Child Development—to establish official liaisons for the revision process.

The Diagnostic Classification Revision Task Force was formed whose members worked both independently and collaboratively, and conferred via conference calls, e-mail, and in-person meetings throughout the 3-year period. Members of the Diagnostic Classification Revision Task Force included the following: Charles H. Zeanah (chair), Alice Carter, Julie Cohen, Helen Egger, Mary Margaret Gleason, Miri Keren, Alicia Lieberman, Kathleen Mulrooney, and Cindy Oser. Robert Emde served as Special Advisor to the Task Force. Helen Egger had served on the Revision Task Force that revised the *Diagnostic Classification of Mental Health and Developmental Disorders of Infancy and Early Childhood* (DC:0–3; ZERO TO THREE, 1994) in 2003–2005. Charles H. Zeanah and Alicia Lieberman served on the original Task Force that developed DC:0–3, and Charles H. Zeanah served as a member of the Childhood and Adolescent Disorders Work Group for the *Diagnostic and Statistical Manual of Mental Disorders* (5th ed.; DSM–5; American Psychiatric Association, 2013). Reflecting on the multidisciplinary nature of infant mental health, the Diagnostic Classification Revision Task Force members included individuals representing the professional disciplines of psychiatry, psychology, pediatrics, nursing, social work, and counseling.

The Diagnostic Classification Revision Task Force was charged with making updates and changes to respond to unresolved issues from DC:0–3R and to capture new findings pertinent to the diagnosis and clinical formulation for infants/young children. The impetus for the revision was that by 2016, more than 10 years had passed since the publication of DC:0–3R. Substantial research on infancy/early childhood psychopathology had been published in that decade; findings from this research were pertinent when revising DC:0–3R. An additional motivation was the publication of DSM–5 in 2013. Although DSM–5 made some attempt to be more developmentally sensitive, it still did not sufficiently capture the range of disorders characteristically seen in infancy/early childhood.

Results of the Users' Survey

To garner feedback from the infant mental health community about DC:0–3R, the Diagnostic Classification Revision Task Force developed and disseminated a web-based survey of 20,000 users of DC:0–3R worldwide in the summer of 2013. Links to the survey instrument were sent to all available DC:0–3R users, including participants in DC:0–3R training sessions; members of the World Association of Infant Mental Health and affiliates; state infant mental health associations and contacts; members of the American Academy of Child and Adolescent Psychiatry Infant and Preschool Committee; members of the Harris Professional Development Network; purchasers of DC:0–3R and related materials; *ZERO TO THREE* journal subscribers; and ZERO TO THREE Board of Directors, staff members, and Academy Fellows. The survey instrument included multiple-choice and open-ended questions dealing with areas of professional discipline and practice (including usual diagnostic procedures), experience with DC:0–3R, as well as thoughts about DC:0–3R's usefulness and thoughts about each Axis of DC:0–3R.

Responses were received from 890 professionals from six continents (80% from the United States). Respondents were highly experienced; were frequent users of DC:0–3R; and included clinicians, providers, researchers, and faculty. Of the respondents, more than half said that they had used DC:0–3R in the past year. Reasons given for not using DC:0–3R included the following: not trained in DC:0–3R, DC:0–3R diagnoses not translatable into *Diagnostic and Statistical Manual of Mental Disorders* (DSM) or *International Classification of Diseases* (ICD) coding, DC:0–3R diagnoses not billable, and DC:0–3R diagnoses not clinically useful in infants/young children.

Respondents suggested adding/defining the following DSM/ICD diagnoses: Pervasive Developmental Disorders, Anxiety Disorders, Other (including Motor Skills Disorders, Communication Disorders, and Intellectual and Developmental Disorders), Reactive Attachment Disorder, Disruptive Behavior Disorders, Attention Deficit Hyperactivity Disorder, and Depressive Disorders.

Survey respondents identified portions of DC:0–3R that needed clarification, highlighted gaps in criteria, and proposed changes in wording. For example, they recognized a need to strengthen the Parent–Infant Relationship Global

Assessment Scale by providing more strengths-based language, more examples, and validation studies. Respondents also identified a need to strengthen Axis III by providing more detail for developmental disorders and conditions and to strengthen Axis V by providing more examples of what regulation looks like at different ages.

Drafting and Further Input

Members of the Diagnostic Classification Revision Task Force systematically reviewed survey results and reviewed new literature pertinent to mental health disorders of infancy/early childhood since DC:0–3R was published in 2005. During biweekly conference calls and face-to-face meetings, the Diagnostic Classification Revision Task Force members began to develop diagnostic criteria.

In an effort to seek additional feedback from the infant mental health community worldwide, proposed revisions in the diagnostic criteria were made available online for public comment in May 2015 and again in October 2015. The Diagnostic Classification Revision Task Force also planned and hosted an update forum in December 2013; a public input session at the World Association of Infant Mental Health Congress in Edinburgh, Scotland, in 2014; and two additional update forums in December 2015 at ZERO TO THREE's National Training Institute. Participants provided feedback at these forums and learned about some of the major changes being deliberated for the revision.

On the basis of this essential feedback, the Diagnostic Classification Revision Task Force gathered specific suggestions about wording of criteria. The Diagnostic Classification Revision Task Force also concentrated on seeking comments from individuals and groups of clinical researchers who were working in areas where differences of opinion among clinicians and researchers existed, as well as comments from individuals and clinical researchers on new disorders. These disorders included Early Atypical Autism Spectrum Disorder, Disorder of Dysregulated Anger and Aggression of Early Childhood, Depressive Disorder of Early Childhood, Inhibition to Novelty Disorder, Overactivity Disorder of Toddlerhood, and Relationship Specific Disorder of Infancy/Early Childhood.

In May 2016, the Diagnostic Classification Revision Task Force previewed a preliminary version of the *DC:0–5: Diagnostic Classification of Mental Health and Developmental Disorders of Infancy and Early Childhood* (DC:0–5™), presenting major aspects of it at the World Association of Infant Mental Health Congress in Prague, Czech Republic.

DC:0–5 is the result of the 3-year process described.

Appendix C
ZERO TO THREE Diagnostic Classification Task Force (DC:0–3) and Revision Task Force (DC:0–3R)

The following list first appeared in the *Diagnostic Classification of Mental Health and Developmental Disorders of Infancy and Early Childhood, Revised Edition* (DC:0–3R; ZERO TO THREE, 2005) and has been updated.

Developers of the original *Diagnostic Classification of Mental Health and Developmental Disorders of Infancy and Early Childhood* (DC:0–3; ZERO TO THREE, 1994) were as follows:

Members

Stanley Greenspan, MD, Chair

Serena Wieder, PhD, Co-Chair

Kathryn Barnard, RN, PhD

Irene Chatoor, MD

Roseanne Clark, PhD

Robert N. Emde, MD

Robert J. Harmon, MD

Alicia F. Lieberman, PhD

Reginald Lourie, MD

Klaus Minde, MD

Joy D. Osofsky, PhD

Sally Provence, MD

Chaya Roth, PhD

Bertram Ruttenberg, MD

Arnold Sameroff, PhD

Rebecca Shahmoon-Shanok, MSW, PhD

Albert J. Solnit, MD

Charles H. Zeanah, MD

Barry Zuckerman, MD

Mark Applebaum, PhD, Research Consultant

Participants, Phase II

Clara Aisenstein, PhD

Marie Anzalone, SciD

Stephen Bennett, MD

Susan Berger, PhD

Barbara Dunbar, PhD

Marguerite Dunitz, MD

Alice Frankel, MD

Eva Gochman, PhD

Peter Gorski, MD

Joyce Hopkins, PhD

Peter Scheer, MD

Madeline Shalowitz, MD

Jean Thomas, MSW, MD

Sylvia Turner, MD

Donna Weston, PhD

Carol Wheeler-Liston, PhD

Molly Romer Witten, PhD

Developers of the DC:0–3R, published in 2005, were as follows:

Members

Robert N. Emde, MD (Chair)

Helen Link Egger, MD

Emily Fenichel, MSW

Antoine Guedeney, MD

Brian K. Wise, MD

Harry H. Wright, MD

Glossary

Adaptive Behavior: The performance of age-expected communication as well as social and daily living skills required for day-to-day adaptive functioning.

Anhedonia: Loss of or markedly diminished pleasure or interest in all, or almost all, activities.

Atopic Disorder: A predisposition toward developing certain allergic hypersensitivity reactions such as eczema and asthma.

Caregiver Accommodations: Modifications made by caregivers to adapt daily routines in response to the infant's/young child's symptoms. Examples include allowing the infant/young child to sleep with the parents even when the parents prefer that the infant/young child sleep alone, avoiding places or situations that the infant/young child finds distressing, allowing the infant/young child to miss school, driving certain routes, removing limit-setting, allowing frequent snacking in a infant/young child with food refusal, removing the infant/young child from child care because of separation distress, and allowing inappropriate behavior.

Caseness: The degree to which an infant's/young child's concerning behaviors are sufficiently serious to warrant clinical attention. In an initial clinical encounter, the practitioner must determine whether the infant's/young child's symptoms constitute a case.

Comorbidity: The existence or presence of more than one disorder or disease at the same time.

Coparenting: An initiative undertaken by two or more individuals to jointly care for and raise children for whom they share responsibility. Coparents may be biological, foster, or adoptive parents (married or divorced, living together or separately); extended family members; or other adult primary caregivers.

Cumulative Risk Hypothesis: The hypothesis that it is the number of risk factors, more than any specific combination of risk factors, that predicts the likelihood of negative outcomes.

Developmental Competence/Competencies: Demonstrated ability to navigate developmentally appropriate or expected social, emotional, cognitive, and behavioral tasks.

Diagnosis: The identification and classification of specific infant/early childhood disorders.

Diathesis: A hereditary or constitutional tendency, predisposition, or vulnerability to a disease or disorder. The diathesis does not cause the disorder but increases risk for the disorder.

Dysphonic: Hoarse or excessively breathy, harsh, or rough speech, although phonation is still possible.

Heterotypic Continuity: A developmental process in which an individual's underlying problems remain consistent but manifest in different behaviors over the course of development. For example, separation anxiety in preschool children predicts social anxiety disorder in school-age children. The anxious diathesis remains constant but the manifestation of the anxiety differs.

Homotypic Continuity: A developmental process in which an individual's behavioral patterns/expressions remain consistent over time. For example, separation anxiety disorder in preschool children predicts separation anxiety in school-age children.

Hyperphonic: Unusually loud speech.

Interoception: Acute awareness of sensations produced by internal body organs (e.g., heartbeat, pulses, or intestinal peristalsis).

Nosology: A classification or list of diseases or disorders.

Parasomnia: A sleep disorder involving abnormal behaviors or physiological events occurring during sleep or sleep–wake transitions. Examples include night (sleep) terrors, sleep walking, and sleep talking.

Parent: Any primary caregiver, whether biological parent or other unrelated adult, who fulfills the parenting role for an infant/young child.

Pediatric Autoimmune Neuropsychiatric Disorders Associated with Streptococcus (PANDAS): A set of disorders in which streptococcal infections trigger rapid onset of obsessive-compulsive behaviors, tics, and anxiety symptoms in young children. Because other agents may also be associated with symptom onset, the disorder is also referred to as Pediatric Autoimmune Neuropsychiatric Disorders (PANS).

Proactive Aggression: Calculated and planned aggression directed toward others with intent to harm or intimidate.

Prodrome: An early symptom (or set of symptoms) that might indicate onset of a disease or disorder before distress or impairment reaches clinical levels.

Proprioceptive Sensation: Sensory feedback reflecting bodily movement and position, including motion of the arms and legs, stretching or contraction of muscles, and so forth.

Reactive Aggression: Aggression directed toward others in response to perceived or actual provocation.

Vestibular Sensation: Sensory feedback reflecting the body's orientation in space (including rotation, balance, and movement).

References

American Psychiatric Association. (1994). *Diagnostic and statistical manual of mental disorders* (4th ed.). Washington, DC: Author.

American Psychiatric Association. (2000). *Diagnostic and statistical manual of mental disorders* (4th ed., text rev.). Washington, DC: Author.

American Psychiatric Association. (2013). *Diagnostic and statistical manual of mental disorders* (5th ed.). Washington, DC: Author.

Ghosh Ippen, C., Noroña, C. R., & Thomas, K. (2012). From tenet to practice: Putting diversity-informed services into action. *ZERO TO THREE, 33*(2), 23–28.

Sarche, M., Tsethlikai, M., Godoy, L., Emde, R., & Fleming, C. (2019). *Cultural perspectives for assessing infants and young children.* Aurora, CO: Anschutz Medical Campus, University of Colorado Denver and Arizona State University, Children's National Health System.

World Health Organization. (1992). *The ICD–10 classification of mental and behavioural disorders: Clinical descriptions and diagnostic guidelines.* Geneva, Switzerland: Author.

ZERO TO THREE. (1994). *Diagnostic classification of mental health and developmental disorders of infancy and early childhood.* Washington, DC: Author.

ZERO TO THREE. (2005). *Diagnostic classification of mental health and developmental disorders of infancy and early childhood* (Rev. ed.). Washington, DC: Author.

Index

failure to speak, 58–60
hearing assessments for unexplained delays, 37
higher expressive than receptive, 20
interrupting or inability to take turns in conversation, 26, 30, 32
RAD and, 129
receptive language abnormalities, 37
regressions and, 117
sleep disorders and, 96
social abnormalities and, 37
social neglect and, 127
speech problems and, 60
stereotyped or repetitive babbling or speech, 17, 22
traumatic mutism and failure to speak, 60
learning disorders, 15, 27, 28
listlessness, 124
low birthweight
ADHD risk and, 29
ASD risk and, 19
EAASD risk and, 24
OADT risk and, 33
Sensory Over-Responsivity Disorder risk and, 44
Tourette's Disorder and, 83

Major Depressive Disorder, 30, 75
medication
anxiety and, 52, 57
assessment of effects, 151
influence on central nervous system functioning, 149
overactivity and, 34
prenatal exposure, 150
sleep problems and, 98
temper dysregulation and, 75
mood disorders, 65–76. *See also specific disorders*
behavioral dysregulation and, 29, 34
caregiver's role in infancy, 65
sleep problems and, 98
motor activity
excessive, 26, 30
repetitive and stereotypies, 17, 20, 22, 24, 80, 81, 82, 83, 84, 87, 127, 128, 129, 131, 132
sluggish, 66, 67
motor delays/deficits, 20, 22. *See also* Developmental Coordination Disorder; movement and physical functioning
ASD and, 17, 20
balance and coordination problems, 27, 38, 39, 40, 41, 129, 132
DCD and, 38–40
DSED and, 131, 132
EAASD and, 22
GDD and, 35–36
motor milestones and, 35, 37, 38, 129
RAD and, 129
social neglect and, 127
visual-motor integration and, 84
Motor or Vocal Tic Disorder, 84–85
age for diagnosis, 85
diagnostic algorithm, 84–85

duration, 85
links to DSM-5 and ICD-10, 85
what to specify, 85
movement and physical functioning
Competency Domain Rating Summary Table, 160
developmental milestones and competency ratings, by age, 163–185

nail biting, 83, 89
National Institute of Mental Health
Research Domain Criteria (RDoC) project, 13
nausea, 59
negative emotionality, 20, 62, 65. *See also* mood disorders
negative self-perceptions, 62
neurodevelopmental disorders, 15–40. *See also specific disorders*
causal factors in, 15
common features of, 15
co-occurences with, 15, 16
environmental neurotoxins and, 15
genetic factors, 15
incidence in males versus females, 15
interventions for, 15
prevalence, industrialized countries, 15
rumination and, 108
sleep problems and, 96
social factors, 15
Nightmare Disorder of Early Childhood, 94
age for diagnosis, 94
diagnostic algorithm, 94
duration, 94
links to DSM-5 and ICD-10, 94
prevalence, 96
night terrors, 93, 96
Night Waking Disorder, 92–93
age for diagnosis, 93
diagnostic algorithm, 92–93
duration, 93
links to DSM-5 and ICD-10, 93
noise-making or noisy behavior, 26, 30
noncompliance, 70, 71, 72

obsessions, 78, 79. *See also* Obsessive Compulsive Disorder
obsessive compulsive and related disorders, 77–88. *See also specific disorders*
cluster with anxiety disorders, 77
genetic factors, 77, 80, 86
major challenge of diagnosing, 77
normative behaviors and, 77, 79
Obsessive Compulsive Disorder (OCD), 77–81
age for diagnosis, 78
associated features supporting diagnoses, 79
caution for abrupt onset, 78, 80
clinically significant behaviors versus normative, 77, 80
comorbidity, 60, 80–81, 83–84
course, 79–80
culture-related diagnostic issues, 80
developmental features, 79
diagnostic algorithm, 78

early childhood depression and, 68

history of procedures, 151

impact of medical conditions on infant's/ young child's experiences, 149

impact of medical conditions on the family, 149–150

markers of health status, 151

medication effects, 151

physical injuries or exposures reflective of the caregiving environment, 151

pregnancy and perinatal complications, 149, 150

recurrent or chronic pain, 151

physiological arousal, 55

pica, 34

associated features supporting diagnoses, 107

comorbidity, 108

course, 108

culture-related diagnostic issues, 108

developmental features, 107

diagnostic algorithm, 106

diagnostic features, 107

differential diagnosis, 108

duration, 106

gender-related diagnostic issues, 108

lack of parental supervision and, 108

links to DSM-5 and ICD-10, 109

medical conditions and, 106

prevalence, 107

risk and prognostic features, 108

what to specify, 106

play

difficulties in engaging, 17, 22

difficulties in reciprocal social games or activities, 16, 21

diminished interest in, 116

fear of new toys, playmates, 61

hyperactivity-impulsivity cluster of ADHD, 26, 31

intrusion into the play of others, 31, 32

reenacting trauma, 115, 117

repetitive use of toys, 17, 22

Posttraumatic Stress Disorder (PTSD), 29, 34, 115–119

age for diagnosis, 114, 116

anxiety disorders and, 53, 57

associated features supporting diagnoses, 117

comorbidity, 76, 118–119

course, 118

culture-related diagnostic issues, 118

defining feature of, 115

developmental features, 117

diagnostic algorithm, 115–116

diagnostic features, 117

differential diagnosis, 118

distinguishing from DDAA, 75

duration, 117

fears of, 63

freezing behavior, 63

gender-related diagnostic issues, 118

links to DSM-5 and ICD-10, 119

physiological reactions, 116

prevalence, 117

risk and prognostic features, 118

sensory response abnormalities and, 41, 42, 44

sleep problems and, 98

specific and nonspecific symptoms, 118

posturing, 20, 83

Prader-Willi syndrome, 102

prenatal conditions and exposures

congenital malformations, 150

genetic abnormalities, 150

injury from maltreatment, 150

prenatal alcohol exposure, 28, 39, 150

prenatal drug exposure, 44

prenatal stress, 74

Sensory Over-Responsivity Disorder risk and, 44

preterm birth, 150

ADHD risk and, 29

ASD risk and, 18

DCD risk and, 39

EAASD risk and, 24

OADT risk and, 33

Sensory Over-Responsivity Disorder risk and, 44

psychomotor retardation, 66, 67

psychosocial stressors, 153–158

cumulative risk hypothesis, 153

examples of, 153

impact of, three factors concerning, 153

Psychosocial and Environmental Stressors, 154–158

pyloric stenosis, 108

Reactive Attachment Disorder (RAD), 21, 24, 126–129

age for diagnosis, 114, 127

associated features supporting diagnoses, 127

comorbidity, 69, 129

core symptoms, 68

course, 128

culture-related diagnostic issues, 128

as a developmental emergency, 128

developmental features, 127

diagnostic algorithm, 126–127

diagnostic features, 127

differential diagnosis, 128–129

duration, 127

gender-related diagnostic issues, 128

links to DSM-5 and ICD-10, 129

prevalence, 127

risk and prognostic features, 128

relationship disorders, 134–138. *See also specific disorders*

Relationship Specific Disorder of Infancy/Early Childhood, 68, 98, 135–138

age for diagnosis, 136

associated features supporting diagnoses, 137

Axis II and, 135, 137, 139

comorbidity, 138

course, 137

culture-related diagnostic issues, 138

developmental features, 137

diagnostic algorithm, 136

diagnostic features, 137